Praise for *Self-Care for Men*

"Any guy who wants to look *and* feel fantastic should own this book."

—Richard Dorment, editor-in-chief of *Men's Health*

"Garrett has a unique grip on men's grooming and how to navigate a crowded field of choices with you in mind. This book contains everything you need to do now for a trusted and healthy life."

—Jim Moore, creative director at large of *GQ*

"Men are notorious for failing to take care of themselves (I know from experience). With Garrett's expert eye and good taste, he reveals how guys can finally practice self-care—and enjoy themselves along the way."

—Michael Sebastian, editor-in-chief of *Esquire*

SELF-CARE

⊰ FOR ⊱

MEN

HOW TO LOOK GOOD
AND FEEL GREAT

GARRETT MUNCE

ADAMS MEDIA

NEW YORK   LONDON   TORONTO   SYDNEY   NEW DELHI

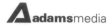

Adams Media
An Imprint of Simon & Schuster, Inc.
57 Littlefield Street
Avon, Massachusetts 02322

Copyright © 2020 by
Simon & Schuster, Inc.

All rights reserved, including the right
to reproduce this book or portions
thereof in any form whatsoever. For
information address Adams Media
Subsidiary Rights Department, 1230
Avenue of the Americas, New York, NY
10020.

First Adams Media hardcover edition
May 2020

ADAMS MEDIA and colophon are
trademarks of Simon & Schuster.

For information about special
discounts for bulk purchases, please
contact Simon & Schuster Special
Sales at 1-866-506-1949 or
business@simonandschuster.com.

The Simon & Schuster Speakers
Bureau can bring authors to your live
event. For more information or to
book an event contact the Simon &
Schuster Speakers Bureau at 1-866-
248-3049 or visit our website at
www.simonspeakers.com.

Interior design by Colleen Cunningham
Interior images by Mathew Wennergren

Manufactured in the United States of
America

10 9 8 7 6 5 4 3 2 1

Library of Congress Cataloging-in-
Publication Data
Names: Munce, Garrett, author.
Title: Self-care for men / Garrett
Munce.
Description: First Adams Media
hardcover edition. | Avon,
Massachusetts: Adams Media, 2020.
Includes index.
Identifiers: LCCN 2019053859 |
ISBN 9781507212547 (hc) | ISBN
9781507212554 (ebook)
Subjects: LCSH: Men--Health and
hygiene--Popular works. | Self-care,
Health--Popular works.
Classification: LCC RA777.8 .M86
2020 | DDC 613/.0423--dc23
LC record available at https://lccn.loc
.gov/2019053859

ISBN 978-1-5072-1254-7
ISBN 978-1-5072-1255-4 (ebook)

Many of the designations used
by manufacturers and sellers to
distinguish their products are
claimed as trademarks. Where those
designations appear in this book and
Simon & Schuster, Inc., was aware of a
trademark claim, the designations have
been printed with initial capital letters.

To Adam,
whose patience with me borders on sainthood,

and Elvira,
whose interest in self-care is unparalleled.

ACKNOWLEDGMENTS

My thanks go to too many people to even begin to list here but I'll try. Thank you to Adam Rathe, for his unwavering support and belief in me. To my parents, who always allowed me space to experiment and create. To my brother, who I hope actually uses all the grooming products I give him. To Ted Stafford, for his energy, unwavering vision, and leadership. To Ross McCammon, who started as an invaluable teacher and ended up a friend. To Jim Moore, whose mentorship has been the most important of my life. To all the brilliant editors who have believed in me: Jim Nelson, Jay Fielden, Rich Dorment, Michael Sebastian, and Stellene Volandes. To David Yi, whose courage and determination are an inspiration. And to all my former and current editors, colleagues, and friends, each of whom have played a part in this book.

CONTENTS

INTRODUCTION

Self-care can mean a lot of things. It can be things you already do, like taking a long shower, working out, or getting your hair cut. But it can also be things like turning off your phone for a few hours, ditching caffeine, and trying meditation. Spend any time on social media and you'll see people doing all manner of things and calling it self-care.

At its core, self-care is doing stuff that makes you feel good. It's focusing on yourself for the sake of wellness. And people are *really* into it. It's become a cultural phenomenon. But it's also more than just feeling good. Self-care helps you stay healthier, live longer, manage stress better, and yes, look better too.

Men are notorious for neglecting themselves. We've been conditioned through years of popular culture and marketing to think of self-care as uniquely female, but self-care is open to everyone, even you. Self-care has no gender, race, class, or sexual orientation. Self-care also isn't something you have to devote all your time to. There are lots of small, easy things you can do to make yourself feel better right away.

Throughout *Self-Care for Men*, you'll find many different ways you can start a self-care practice. Whether you are new to self-care or just looking for some fresh options this book will show you a variety of ways you can care for yourself without breaking the bank or giving up your whole day. Your personal routine can be simple, like applying moisturizer regularly or washing your hair properly. You can start by taking supplements, getting more sleep, or even getting a tattoo. The most important thing is to start thinking of these things as part of self-care. Personal grooming, for instance, is necessary, but it's also a way to show your body you care for it; it makes you feel good, inside and out. That's one of the keys to self-care: Sometimes when you look good, you feel even better.

Some of the things in this book might surprise you. Blow drying your hair can really be self-care, you might ask? Yes, it can. Crystals can actually make you feel better? Yup, they do. Does having a houseplant really affect your mood? It can, and there's actually science behind it.

The bottom line is that no one is going to stand over you and force you to do any of this, but if you give it a shot, you'll be surprised at how great self-care can make you feel. Now, open your mind and let's get started.

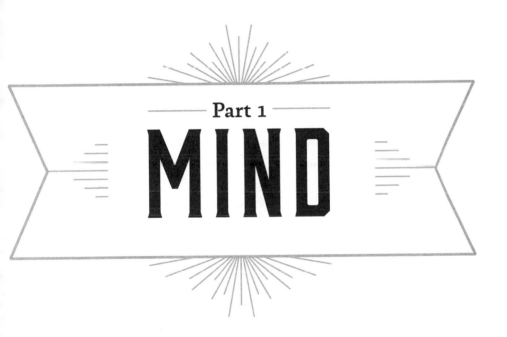

Part 1

MIND

You've probably observed on social media that a lot of self-care focuses on relaxing your body and reducing stress and anxiety. That's because pent-up stress and anxiety can have very real effects on your body. They can also have negative effects on your mind. But people tend to focus so much on their outsides that they neglect their insides, especially what's going on between their ears.

Some of the things you'll find in this part are straightforward, like how meditation can help you stay calm. That may not be news to you, whether or not you've tried it for yourself. Other things you find in this part might surprise you, like how taking your self-care routine on the road with you is as much a mental practice as it is a physical one. Think about it for a second: So much anxiety comes from outside forces, so why should your self-care routine only be made of things that you do at home? You need tools to deal with stress at all times of your life, especially when you're not at home.

Ultimately, we're talking about mental health, and that's important for everyone. Self-care is one of the most important tools you have to improve your mental health. But remember that it's not the only tool. Self-care can take you far, but if you think you might have a serious mental health issue, seek professional help. For all those other times you feel burned out or beaten down, here are some solutions.

MEDITATION: NOT JUST FOR BUDDHA

When you hear the word "meditation" you probably think of a Buddhist monk sitting on top of a mountain. In your head, this dude has been there for days, maybe even years, and is so calm he barely moves. He's enlightened, and he's totally unattainable.

In reality, meditation is much simpler than moving to a monastery in the Himalayas. Anyone can meditate and many more people than you'd probably expect do it. It doesn't mean they're sitting at home on a Friday night chanting the word "om." Meditation can be simple, quick, and done anywhere. Think of your mind as a muscle (not your brain, but your *mind*) and meditation as the workout you do to make it stronger.

What Is Meditation?

Simply put, the practice of meditation is clearing your mind. Doing this means focusing on your awareness and training your mind to focus on one thing in an effort to clear out all the other noise. The goal is to achieve a state of calm for a sustained period of time.

Anyone who has tried to meditate before knows that it's much harder than it sounds. Many beginners get frustrated because they are having a hard time clearing their minds and not getting caught up in their thoughts. This frustration leads them to abandon meditation and say it's "too hard." Many teachers, however, say the secret of meditation is that it's not easy for anyone. That's why it's called a practice. It takes skill and experience to be able to totally clear your mind, and many people who have meditated for years still can't do it. The practice of meditating is in the experience; meditating successfully is a journey, not a destination.

Why Do It?

Meditation is an ancient practice used across cultures for centuries. Recently, scientific studies have found that meditation has measurable effects on both your body and mind. It has been shown to lower blood pressure, lower your heart rate, and improve the blood circulation throughout your body. Many meditation practices focus on breath work, so it also physically slows down your breathing and allows more oxygen to circulate in your bloodstream.

Mentally, meditation has been shown to decrease anxiety, lower stress, elevate mood, and reduce cortisol levels in the brain. Studies have shown that people with consistent meditation practices benefit from these effects even when they're not meditating. It has been shown to allow practitioners to better manage their anxiety and stress in the long run.

Types of Meditation

Meditation is exercise for your brain, and just like working out, there are a lot of different ways to do it. There is no one-size-fits-all solution. These are some of the most common meditation styles.

Mindfulness

This is one of the most popular forms of meditation and is built on the assumption that you will not be able to completely clear your mind. That's okay! Mindfulness meditation encourages you to acknowledge thoughts as they come and let them pass through your mind without judgment. It usually involves focusing on a specific thing, like your breath, to help divert focus away from your thoughts.

Transcendental

This form of meditation is arguably the most popular worldwide and the most scientifically studied. It's popular among celebrities (the Beatles were fans and so are David Lynch, Jerry Seinfeld, and Ellen DeGeneres) and is a more structured form of meditation than some others. It involves focusing on a mantra (a word or series of words that you repeat aloud to help focus your thoughts). Usually, to learn Transcendental Meditation, you must seek out an accredited teacher.

Mantra

As mentioned previously, a mantra is a word or series of words that are repeated to help focus your mind. By focusing on the words, the theory is that your mind is able to clear itself of other thoughts more easily. Some people find this type of meditation helpful because it provides you something to do. If you find focusing on your breath too difficult or sitting with your own thoughts too scary, starting with mantra meditation might be good for you.

Guided

Thanks to the popularity of meditation, new apps and classes are popping up everywhere. Most of these use guided meditation, in which a voice or teacher guides you through the meditation process, either by taking you on a journey to visualize in your head or simply talking you through the process of breath work and mindfulness. This type is especially good for novices, as they might have a hard time sitting in silence for a sustained period of time.

Movement

One of the biggest hurdles some people face when beginning a meditation practice is sitting for a long period of time. Whether it's a physical response like joint pain or more of a restlessness, those people may be better suited to movement meditation. This type allows you to move through a series of poses, like yoga, or any sort of other sustained and/or repetitive action, like going on a walk or even cleaning your house. The goal isn't to raise your heart rate but instead allow your body to go on autopilot and let your mind focus on itself.

How to Meditate for Beginners

No matter what form of meditation you choose, the biggest hurdle can be actually starting. Many people get intimidated by meditation itself and think that if they can't sit in silence for half an hour that they won't be able to meditate. Remember that a meditation practice is about going through the process, not about doing it perfectly from the very beginning. Be kind to yourself and allow yourself to be uncomfortable. There is no such thing as failure in meditation. To get started, here are some simple steps:

1. Sit or lie down in a comfortable position. You don't have to sit in the lotus position. Choose a comfortable chair or maybe a meditation cushion on the floor. Remember that you want to be comfortable enough that you can stay in that position for about 20 minutes but not so comfortable that you fall asleep.
2. Close your eyes. If keeping your eyes closed for a long period of time is difficult, or you think you might get distracted, use an eye mask to cover your eyes.

3. If you're first starting out, don't try to control your breath. Breathe naturally and deeply.

4. As you're breathing, focus on how that breath feels in your body. Notice how the air feels going into your nostrils or mouth, how your lungs feel as they fill up with air, and how your rib cage expands with the air. Try to keep your focus on your breath. As your mind wanders (and it will; there's no shame in it), try to bring your attention back to your breath.

5. Start slow and do this for about 3–5 minutes. Try doing this every day, and as you get more practiced gradually increase the amount of time of each session. Eventually you want to get to about 15–20 minutes for each meditation session.

THERE'S AN APP FOR THAT

Thanks to modern technology, it's never been easier to start a meditation practice. There are hundreds of smartphone apps that help you experiment with meditation styles, track your progress, and even help you quickly relax on the go or at the office. Most of these apps have guided meditations that are ideal for beginners. They make it easy to just pop in your headphones and meditate for a few minutes wherever you are. Some even have specific meditations for different goals like sleep, focus, stress relief, and happiness. The differences in these meditations are subtle, but the ultimate goal is the same: making meditation easy and accessible.

STICK IT TO THE MAN: WHAT ACUPUNCTURE DOES

To the uninitiated, acupuncture can seem like a lot of hocus pocus. You've seen the pictures of people lying on beds with needles stuck all over their bodies. How could that possibly help with anything? The reality is that acupuncture is an ancient remedy used for centuries in Chinese medicine and has been scientifically proven to help not only physical ailments but mental ones as well.

In order to understand how acupuncture works, you have to understand how traditional Chinese medicine views the body. Think of the body like a road map. There are different channels called meridians that run all over the body. These meridians are like roads for energy. Some are big; think of them as the highways. Others are small, like side streets or paths. All of them work together to keep energy flowing through all the areas of the body. When everything is running smoothly, energy is able to reach where it needs to go in order to keep everything on track. But when there are blockages, like traffic jams, energy can get diverted or trapped. In Chinese medicine, this is what causes pain (and a host of other issues).

Acupuncture is a way to clear these blockages. Traditional Chinese medicine says that there are specific points along this complex meridian road map that, when activated, can open up passageways and allow energy to flow through. Acupuncture, the practice where tiny stainless steel needles are stuck into your skin superficially, is a way of activating these pressure points.

What It Can Do for You

Typically, the conversations around acupuncture center on physical ailments. It's been found to be an effective tool in relieving all sorts of pain from muscle and joint ailments to even chronic inflammation inside the body. It's used for chronic heart issues, breathing problems, gastrointestinal issues, and even fatigue. It can also be used to address superficial issues like skin and hair problems by promoting blood flow to the surface.

Less discussed is the ability of acupuncture to treat non-physical ailments as well. Studies have shown that acupuncture can help alleviate anxiety, depression, fear, and even addiction. A popular use for acupuncture is smoking cessation. It has also been found to be an effective treatment for more serious anxiety disorders like post-traumatic stress disorder and social anxiety disorder.

Choosing a Practitioner

Acupuncture is a highly specialized practice that many spend years, even decades, studying. Choosing an acupuncturist should be a careful process. Some will have medical degrees, but that shouldn't be your only indicator. Look for specific certifications in acupuncture and Chinese medicine. You may want to search for terms like "homeopath" or "naturopath" as well; these holistic doctors will sometimes be trained in acupuncture as well as herbalism and other forms of "alternative" medicine.

Do your research. Acupuncture may seem simple to the layman, but a lot can go wrong if it's not done properly or the facility isn't clean. Check online review sites. Read every review and pay close attention to the average review, not just the very positive or very negative. You may also want to ask your general doctor for a recommendation. Many medical doctors are starting to recommend acupuncture as a supplement to Western medical treatments and have pre-screened networks to draw upon. Finally, remember to trust your gut. Just because you go to one person for your first appointment doesn't mean you're locked in. If you don't vibe with them, try another provider.

What to Expect from Your First Appointment

The biggest thing to remember when going to your first acupuncture appointment is to treat it like any other doctor visit. Acupuncture is a medical specialty, so treat it as such.

1. Your first appointment will start with a consultation. The provider will ask you in detail about the ailments you are hoping to treat with acupuncture. Be honest and treat this like a checkup with your general doctor. It doesn't do you any good to not be forthcoming with everything. They may ask you questions about your diet, your lifestyle, your stress levels, and previous and current medical conditions.
2. Next, your provider will likely do some evaluating. They'll do some things you're probably used to, like feel your pulse and take a look at your tongue and mouth. They'll also poke and prod you to see what areas have pain or inflammation. They may also do some things you're not used to, like look at the color of your face, inspect your feet, and even use tools like crystals or a pendulum to access energy flow.
3. The acupuncturist will then let you know what their plan of action is. They'll let you know what areas of the body they will focus the needles on. Keep in mind that many acupuncture

points are far away from the point of physical pain. For instance, pain in your elbow might mean putting some needles in your feet. You're not expected to understand this complicated system on the first visit, so sit back and go with the flow. If you need to remove any clothing, they'll tell you.

As an example, here's a look at the acupuncture points for stomach pain.

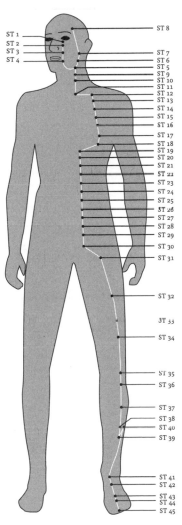

4. You'll lie back on a table and relax. The practitioner will then start inserting needles into your skin. The process is superficial, and the needles are very small, so you may not feel anything at all. If you do, that's okay, and the acupuncturist will guide you through it.

5. Once the needl es are inserted, you'll be asked to relax for usually around 20 minutes while the needles go to work. The practitioner might dim the lights, put on some soothing music, and maybe even leave the room to help you relax. If you fall asleep, that's normal.

6. Once the session is over, the acupuncturist will remove the needles. Depending on what ailment you are hoping to

treat, they may leave small tacks (called seeds) on certain points. You won't feel them, but they are meant to keep the energy flow to those points open even after the session is over.

7. After an acupuncture session, some people feel relaxed and others feel energetic. It really depends on what was being treated in the session.

NOT JUST PINS AND NEEDLES

Depending on who you go to for acupuncture, they may incorporate other similar treatments into your session. These are some of the most common.

- **Acupressure:** Similar to acupuncture, this is based on the meridian map and pressure points of your body. Instead of using needles, acupressure uses massage and pressure.
- **Reiki:** This is a form of energy manipulation, where the practitioner helps move and rebalance your energy with their hands. They may not even touch your body in the process, but instead move their hands just above the surface.
- **Reflexology:** Based on the idea that different pressure points in your hands and feet are connected to internal organs, this may feel closer to a hand or foot massage.
- **Cupping:** This practice is particularly useful for physical pain management and is when cups are placed on certain parts of the body to create suction and manipulate energy flow. It's also believed that it can aid in detoxing.

TIME MANAGEMENT AS SELF-CARE

Everyone's had it, that feeling that there is too much to do and not enough time. You've maybe even said the words "there's not enough time in the day." You're not alone. The biggest source of anxiety for many men is their work—more particularly, that there is too much work to be done and not enough time to do it.

Here's the bad news: It's impossible to create more time. The good news is that you can learn to use this time more wisely. Time management is one of the most important skills a man can learn to not only be more productive but also reduce his stress and anxiety. In short: Time management is self-care.

It's simple, really. The more time you have, the less stressed you'll be. It goes beyond that too. If you manage your time wisely, you'll have more time to focus on yourself. If you're thinking, "Who has time to take a bath?" or "I can't possibly sleep 8 hours every day," then consider time management your first step to self-care.

How Time Management Can Help Anxiety

People who are not good at time management sometimes have higher rates of anxiety, but the daunting task of "getting it all done" on a daily basis is something everyone feels in today's busy world. The way effective time management helps ease anxiety and stress is somewhat indirect. When you feel you have so much to do that you can't possibly get it all done, that insurmountable feeling creates anxiety. It can also lead to procrastination, which creates more anxiety because you feel guilty for not getting stuff done. More practically, if you have too much to do, you may forgo sleep, which can be detrimental to your physical and mental health (turn to Part 2 to find out how).

Alleviating anxiety through time management doesn't mean you have to check off your entire to-do list every day, but it does mean doing your best. It can also mean giving yourself permission to be flexible. Being too rigid can be a detriment to time management. Like most things in life, it's about balance, and finding the right balance for you can make a big difference in your stress level.

Time Management Tips

Not all time management skills work for everyone. You may need to experiment to see what works best for you. These are some good places to start.

Make a To-Do List the Day Before

Every evening, make a list of tasks you want to accomplish the next day. The most important thing is that you be realistic and don't set yourself up for failure. Prioritize what you need to do higher on the list and what you want to do lower. Doing this the night before allows you to start the day with a game plan instead of waking up overwhelmed. At the end of the day, move any unchecked tasks to the next day's list.

Use a Calendar

Writing things down works. If you write something down, like an appointment or deadline, you are less likely to forget about it. Use your calendar for big events like trips, presentations, and deadlines. Also use it for smaller things, like setting goals for yourself or when to make an important phone call. You probably use a calendar at work, but you should have one for your personal life too (ideally the same one). Consolidating the places you keep track of things will only help you. Use the calendar to help break up larger tasks into smaller, actionable items that you can put on your daily to-do list.

Make Things Habits

For smaller things that you want to do every day, like taking vitamins or creating a to-do list, you have to do them consistently. Some studies say that forming a habit takes an average of two months of consistent activity. It's different for everyone, but forming habits can take some of the pressure off remembering to do small things. Consider what your goals are in forming the habit and then make a point to do it every day consistently. Make it easy on yourself. If you want to take vitamins every day, for instance, keep them by your coffee machine so you remember to take them first thing.

Limit Multitasking

Multitasking, or being able to do multiple things at once, is usually considered valuable in the workplace (how many of you have "good multitasker" on your resume?). But in terms of time management, it can be a detriment. Instead, try to focus on one task at a time. It will allow you to finish that task more quickly so you can check it off your list and move on. This also might mean limiting distractions, like turning off the TV if you're working from home or wearing noise-canceling headphones in a noisy office.

Practice Time Blocking

Time blocking can be a useful tool for people who struggle with distraction and multitasking. It means scheduling blocks of time in which you focus on one single task until it's done. These tasks can be large or small, but the most important thing is that you allow enough time to truly focus on the task at hand. Be realistic: If a task is going to take you longer than an hour, schedule accordingly. The idea here is to finish tasks effectively, not rush through them. For larger tasks, break them up into multiple blocks and schedule smaller tasks or breaks between them.

Take Regular (Short) Breaks

About those breaks: You should be taking them. Especially when you're tackling a more time-consuming task, schedule in short breaks every so often. Constructive breaks should be around 15 minutes to allow you time to get up from your desk, walk around a bit, maybe drink a glass of water. You want to be refreshed and ready to start again when you sit down. If you have a problem with procrastination, limit your breaks to a smaller time frame to help decrease the likelihood of distraction.

Allow for Flexibility

It's a fact of life that things will always pop up. When this happens (like an urgent task from your boss or an unexpected family commitment), don't stress about it. Look at your to-do list and see what you can de-prioritize in favor of this new task. You may need to consistently change around the priority of tasks throughout the day. That's fine too. Just make sure you're doing it because something requires your attention, not because you are putting it off.

Learn to Say No

People who take on too much work tend to be more overwhelmed and stressed out. That's a fact. Many of us have issues turning down tasks, especially if we are freelancers or work for ourselves. When presented with a new task, take a serious look at your to-do list. Can you realistically take this on without sacrificing something else? If the answer is no, you need to consider turning it down. It can be hard at first, but learning to say no to something can have a positive impact on your stress level.

Prioritize Yourself

In today's world, everyone puts so much focus on their jobs and other things that take their focus away from themselves. Loving your work is not a bad thing, but when it becomes all-consuming it can cause stress and anxiety to go through the roof. When scheduling your time and making your to-do list, always reserve some time for something you want to do. This could mean scheduling around a favorite workout class at the gym or leaving enough time at night to do your skincare routine. Make sure that each day includes something that makes you feel good in the name of self-care.

THE MOST IMPORTANT PART OF YOUR DAY

You may not think you're a morning person, but your brain probably thinks differently. Some studies have shown that the brain is more active and creative right after sleep than at any other time of the day. Studies also show that your energy levels and brain activity are best right when you wake up. This means that the first few hours of the day can be your most productive. Utilizing those first hours (particularly the first 1 to 3 hours) of your day, you may find that you have more time during the rest of the day to watch puppy videos on *Twitter*.

SELF-CARE ON THE MOVE

The downfall of many conversations around self-care is that they focus too much on things you do at home, but most of us don't actually spend all that much time there. Think about it: You're spending most of your day at the office, you're in your car or on public transportation all the time, or you're traveling for work or for vacation. The amount of time you're realistically spending in your own space is probably fairly low compared to how often you're on the go.

So what does that mean for your self-care? You're not likely to stop in the middle of a meeting and meditate on the conference room table. Building a good self-care routine that you can do at home is one thing, but building one that you can do anywhere is another.

Having a self-care toolbox that you can draw upon wherever you are is important. Anxiety and stress don't happen in a vacuum. Things that you encounter in the world every day—like demanding bosses, bad drivers, traffic jams, long lines at the grocery store—all have an impact on your stress and anxiety levels. Sometimes they can build up so much that they become overwhelming. If you expect to be able to run home and take a bath every time you get stressed, you need to reconceptualize your self-care routine.

Many of the main aspects of self-care remain in place no matter where you are. Checking in with yourself is possible. So is calming yourself down when you feel anxious or stressed. It could be as simple as doing some controlled breathing or popping on some headphones and listening to a meditation app.

Why It Matters

Most of this book discusses how self-care can help chill you out, but many people have increased anxiety when they're out in the world. Do you have a problem with road rage? Are you an anxious flyer? Do you get freaked out by crowds? Self-care can help with all of those things. A constructive self-care practice will be useful wherever you are and especially in stressful situations (which don't always happen at home).

How to Build a Mobile Self-Care Practice

The most important thing with any self-care practice is to plan ahead. This goes for whether you're getting in the car to go to work or packing for an extended vacation. Think about the self-care tools you enjoy at home and how they could translate to where you are going. It's not always as simple as packing a sheet mask in your carry-on bag, but it could be. Plan ahead and make sure you always have at least one self-care tool at the ready should the need arise.

On Vacation

Even on the most relaxing vacation, it's possible to get overwhelmed and stressed. As you're planning your trip, include activities that are meant specifically to promote self-care.

- **Meditate:** Keeping a meditation app on your phone can help you keep up your practice wherever you are.
- **Go for walks:** Just like at home, moderate activity will help promote blood flow and increase your endorphins.

- **Get into nature:** No matter where you're going, plan activities that will get you out into nature. The positive effects have been proven (turn to Part 6 for more on this).
- **Take your journal:** If you use journaling as a self-care tool, don't leave home without it.
- **Plan a spa visit:** Spas can be found all over the world, so no matter where you are, consider visiting one (even if it's just in your hotel).
- **Allow yourself to splurge:** Even if you're traveling on a budget, plan on splurging on one thing. This could be a fancy dinner or paying for a checked bag. Stressing about money the whole trip will only cause anxiety.

In the Car

Spending time in your car is a reality of life for most people, whether it's driving to and from work or just running errands. Turning your car into a self-care sanctuary can be a huge help in managing stress.

- **Don't take work calls in the car:** Consider your car a safe space apart from the pressures of work. Leave any work calls for when you're done driving.
- **Turn your phone on silent:** Hearing your phone ding with every new email or text message won't just cause anxiety but will also distract you from watching the road.
- **Listen to a podcast:** Soothing music might relax you, but it could also make you sleepy. Instead, opt for a podcast since the sounds of talking can be just as soothing.
- **Practice breathing exercises:** No one is going to suggest you try to meditate while you're driving, but using controlled breathing to manage stress can help you calm down, especially when you're stuck in a traffic jam or feel road rage coming on.

- **Use aromatherapy to your advantage:** Getting an air freshener for your car might seem cliché, but using a car diffuser with natural essential oils like lavender can help you maintain your cool and keep you chilled out.

At the Office

Most people spend at least 40 hours a week at work, many people more than that, so figuring out self-care practices you can do at the office can help make it a little more tolerable. They'll also help you manage the stress that comes with your job.

- **Get up from your desk:** Getting up from your desk every so often (some say as much as once an hour) can help keep blood flowing and your energy high.
- **Declutter your space:** It's been said that a messy desk is the sign of a messy mind. Keeping your area clutter-free can help decrease anxiety.
- **Get a plant:** You might not be able to get out into nature during the workday, but keeping a plant at your desk can have a positive effect on your mood.
- **Scent your space:** Chances are you can't light a candle in your office without arousing suspicion (or setting off the fire alarm), but using a small diffuser with essential oils can have a positive effect on your mood.
- **Focus on your strengths:** It's easy to get caught up in the stress and negativity of others when you're working in the same office. When you feel down, remind yourself of the things you are good at and doing right. You might even want to keep a list at your desk and look at it whenever you're feeling stressed out.
- **Breathing exercises:** Sure, you could pop on some headphones and turn on a meditation app. But if you can't, 1 minute of deep breathing will help calm anxiety.

On a Plane

Many people would classify themselves as nervous flyers. Even if you don't, long flights can be stressful (screaming kids, tight seats, weird smells). Self-care can help get you through any flight unscathed.

- **Stretch:** Especially on long flights, it's important to get up every so often and move around the cabin. You don't have to do jumping jacks in the aisle, but walking a bit will help blood circulate.
- **Get noise-canceling headphones:** At the very least they'll help drown out that baby crying a few rows in front of you. At best, they'll let you listen to your meditation app in peace.
- **Bring healthy food:** Airplane food is just the worst, right? Bringing your own healthy food can keep you from feeling gross even after you get off the plane.
- **Skin care:** Skin can dry out quickly in the recycled air of a plane. Bring a cleansing wipe, moisturizer, and face mist to keep your skin feeling fresh. Bonus points for a sheet mask.
- **In-flight massage:** Especially on long flights, using small massaging balls to relieve tension on your feet and neck can help relieve pain and relax you in the process.

HOW TO BUILD A SELF-CARE GO BAG

Keeping a self-care-focused travel kit primed and ready for travel can not only help alleviate stress in the air or in the car, but also take the stress out of packing. Find a small dopp kit and keep it packed with self-care essentials so you can just grab and go. Some things to keep in it:

- Your favorite sheet mask
- Lavender essential oil in a roller ball
- A hydrating face mist
- Some high-end, good-smelling hand cream
- Natural sleep aids like melatonin supplements
- Healing ointment for chapped skin and lips
- Cleansing face wipes
- A travel-sized container of your favorite cologne
- CBD tincture or gummies

DITCH THE CAFFEINE: FIVE WAYS TO GET ENERGY WITHOUT COFFEE

What's a section about caffeine doing in a book about self-care, you might be asking, much less in a part about your brain? It's actually pretty simple. How many times have you said to someone, "Don't talk to me before I've had my coffee"? Coffee is such a big part of so many people's lives that we give it more power than it deserves. You might drink it every morning to wake up. You might drink another cup in the afternoon when you're feeling sluggish. You might think of caffeine as a necessity in your daily life, but many also consider it one of the most common (and socially acceptable) drugs. That's because while it does have an impact on your physical body, it can also have an impact on your brain.

Why Caffeine Can Be Bad for Your Brain

By textbook definition, you cannot get addicted to caffeine. However, the reason some people consider it a drug is because of how it affects your brain. Moderate doses of caffeine have been shown to increase alertness and brain function; too much caffeine can have the opposite effect. It can cause brain fog and even increase anxiety. It can make mood changes happen faster, make highs and lows more extreme, and in some cases, increase paranoia. And because these beneficial changes in alertness are short-term, we can convince ourselves that we need more and more if it to get the desired effects.

While experts say you cannot get addicted to caffeine, you can go through withdrawal symptoms if you are used to having it. Withdrawal symptoms can include jitters, headaches, and fatigue. They can also include difficulty concentrating, mood swings, and anxiety. Basically, sustained caffeine use can make the very things you are hoping to avoid by drinking caffeine worse, and withdrawal from caffeine can bring them on harder.

What Does Caffeine Have to Do with Self-Care?

It's simple really. The goal of self-care is to reduce stress, decrease anxiety, and help you deal with the demands of daily life in a more constructive way. If caffeine has a negative impact on your emotional health and may actually increase anxiety by extension, it may benefit you to consider an alternative. Not to mention, excessive coffee consumption has been linked to actual health issues like acid reflux, digestive issues, and even heart disease. Keep in mind that there are some benefits to caffeine and coffee, but it depends on how much coffee you are drinking a day. Experts say that anything more than two cups can actually be detrimental to your health in the long run. And isn't self-care about promoting health?

Five Coffee Replacements

Replacing your daily cup(s) of coffee doesn't mean that you have to forgo caffeine altogether, especially if you're concerned about withdrawal symptoms. What constitutes a positive replacement to coffee is usually the amount of caffeine in it. Some also have more beneficial ingredients, like antioxidants, than are typically found in coffee.

1. **Green tea:** Tea, which is made from brewing the leaves of a plant, still has some caffeine, but is also loaded with antioxidants and other nutrients that are beneficial for your body.
2. **Golden milk:** Golden milk is the common term for a concoction made from almond milk, turmeric, and other spices like cinnamon. There is no caffeine, but if you're looking for the rich feeling of your favorite latte, this will come close.
3. **Hot water with lemon:** Many people claim that drinking hot water with lemon right when you wake up helps awaken your bodily systems and aid in digestion. There is no caffeine, but the vitamin C in the lemon gives your system a jolt.
4. **Apple cider vinegar:** You should never drink apple cider vinegar straight up, but diluting one or two tablespoons in a glass of water has been said to promote digestion and help regulate blood levels. There is no caffeine in this either.
5. **Kombucha:** This drink is usually made from fermenting bacteria and yeast in tea. These bacteria have a gut-healthy probiotic quality and through the fermentation process develop a high level of antioxidants. There is usually no caffeine in kombucha, but some varieties have a small amount of alcohol thanks to the fermentation process.

Other Ways to Boost Your Energy

It is possible to get a jolt of energy without turning to coffee for help. Most of it involves small lifestyle changes that help you feel more energetic and stay that way longer.

Get More Sleep
Getting at least 7 hours of sleep a night can help you feel more alert and focused during the day.

Change Your Diet
Increasing the antioxidants in your diet, which can be found in many fruits and vegetables, can help your body run more efficiently and give you more energy.

Go for Walks
When you feel tired, get up and move around a little bit. It could be as simple as walking around the block or your office. Getting your heart beating and blood flowing helps more oxygen reach other parts of your body.

Take a Power Nap
Not everyone has the chance to take a nap in the middle of the day, but studies have shown that a short, 15-minute nap can leave you feeling more energetic.

Use Adaptogenic Herbs
This specific family of herbs can help decrease inflammation in your body and increase energy levels. For more about them, turn to Part 2.

COFFEE OBSESSION BY THE NUMBERS

You're not the only one who's obsessed with coffee. Coffee consumption might as well be an official American pastime.

- 63—percentage of Americans who drink at least one cup of coffee daily
- 3.1—how many cups of coffee the average American drinks per day
- 66 billion—how many cups of coffee are consumed in the US per year
- 47,840—how many cups of coffee the average full-time office worker will consume during their career
- 24—how many minutes a day the average person spends making and drinking coffee
- 20—percent by which the sale of specialty coffees increased in 2018

Statistics from the National Coffee Association

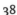

WE NEED TO TALK ABOUT MENTAL HEALTH

It's simple: Some of the biggest issues people face in modern society are stress and anxiety. These things, when left unchecked, can have wide-ranging consequences on your physical health, but also on your mental state. It's been found that reducing stress can help you be happier, have more fulfilling relationships, and live a fuller life. It's also been found that neglecting your physical and mental health (i.e., not engaging in self-care activities) can result in serious illness, both physical and mental. Psychologists often assess someone's inability to perform self care activities, such as bathing and brushing their teeth, as an indicator for things like anxiety disorders and clinical depression.

On Masculinity and Mental Health

Some have said we're in the middle of a male mental health crisis; others have noted that we're currently experiencing a crisis of masculinity. The two are not mutually exclusive. According to the organization Mental Health America, around six million men are affected by depression each year. However, men are much less likely to seek out mental healthcare than women. This is because many men are taught to not talk openly about their feelings. You know that phrase "the strong, silent type"? It's what men are taught to aspire to, and it can be detrimental to their mental health. Not to mention the fact that most men still view showing emotion, especially crying, as a feminine quality.

This means that thousands of mental health issues in men go undiagnosed each year. Admitting that you care about your mental health, or that you need to do something about it, is not an admission of weakness. In fact, taking steps to improve your mental health can be one of the strongest things a man can do.

How Self-Care Can Support Mental Health

Many men's mental health issues can be linked to stress, and they often come from work. More men report that stress from their jobs affects their mental state even when they are not at work. Men also say that anxiety about their jobs can have a detriment to their ability to enjoy life outside of work. Developing a positive self-care routine can be a useful tool in learning to deal with this stress. It can also be a good outlet for aggression and anxiety.

Similarly, just like a positive self-care routine can help you get in touch with your body, it can also help you get in touch with your emotions. Some people with depression or the victims of abuse have a hard time taking care of their physical bodies. Self-care can help you get in touch with your body and can also promote a positive self-image. It's been shown that people who can care for themselves well are better able to manage stress but also care for others more effectively.

Tips for Promoting Mental Health

Promoting your own mental health, and making it a priority, takes a bit of awareness and some small changes in your routine. If you worry that mental health is an issue for you, seek the help of a professional.

Don't Isolate Yourself

Spending time alone can be good for recharging your mind and body, but too much of it can actually be a detriment to your mental health. It's been shown that people with strong interpersonal relationships are usually happier than people who don't have any. If you notice you're isolating yourself, make an effort to meet up with a friend or accept a social invitation you would have otherwise turned down.

Keep a Journal

One of the reasons so many men go undiagnosed with mental health issues is that they don't want to talk about their emotions. If you're unable to talk to someone, keep a journal instead. Writing down what you are thinking and feeling allows you to process emotions constructively instead of keeping them locked inside and can lead to higher emotional understanding.

Set Aside Time Each Day to Focus on Yourself

Taking care of yourself can seem unimportant when you're stressed about other things going on, but finding time each day to do something that makes you happy can make a huge difference in your mental well-being. It could be as simple as reading a chapter of a book or going to the gym. What you choose to do isn't important as long as it makes you happy.

Practice Gratitude

Studies have shown that positive thinking actually has an impact on your outlook and ability to deal with stress. Gratitude practices are simple and effective ways to increase positive thinking. Some people keep gratitude journals, where they write down what they are thankful for, and others choose to say affirmations in the mirror. The most important thing is that it gives you the ability to recognize the positive things in your life.

Put Down Your Smartphone

Excessive smartphone use can make isolation from other people easier. It can also increase anxiety and stress in your life if you're constantly checking your work email or reading the news on *Twitter*. Find a few minutes a day to take a break from your phone. This could mean turning it off earlier at night or leaving it at home while you go for a walk. Encourage other members of your family to do the same so you can interact face to face instead.

Get Moving

In Part 2, you'll learn that exercise can be a form of self-care. The same goes for its impact on mental health. Moderate exercise, even just going on a short walk, can help raise endorphins and other good hormones in your brain that promote happiness and stress reduction.

Practice Forgiveness

You know all those little things that piss you off throughout the day? They build up in your mind and create anxiety that has nowhere to go. Instead of getting angry when someone cuts you off in their car, for instance, let it go. Forgiveness can also mean forgiving yourself. Did you make a mistake on a report? Don't beat yourself up about it. Tell yourself you won't make the same mistake again and move on.

Download an App

In addition to other apps that have been discussed in this book, there are also apps to help promote mental health. Cognitive puzzles and "brain teasers" can help strengthen your thinking and problem-solving skills. Others, like therapy apps, can help connect you to professionals if you need someone to talk to. Using these apps is easy and portable, so consider making them part of your mental self-care routine.

Find a Community

Finding a community of like-minded people, whether in real life or online, can make a big difference in your happiness and self-esteem. Look for message boards and online forums where people are discussing things you identify with. Look for ads in your local community for mixers and groups for people like you. Join a recreational sports team or a book club. Finding even just one other person you can talk to can make a huge difference.

A NOTE ON THERAPY

It used to be thought that going to therapy meant something was wrong with you or that you were "crazy." Well, we don't use that word anymore, and we shouldn't think that way about therapy. At its most basic level, therapy is a safe space where you are able to talk about things with an impartial party that you otherwise might not feel comfortable voicing. It can also provide perspective on issues in your life that you might not know how to deal with. Sure, seeking out therapy for a specific issue like addiction or depression is important, but you don't need a reason like that to start going. If you're wary, you don't even have to tell anyone. And thanks to modern therapy apps, you might not even have to leave your house. So there really is no excuse.

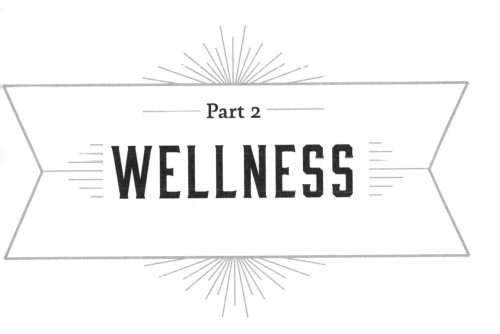

Part 2

WELLNESS

In the conversation around self-care, a lot of emphasis is placed on doing things to the outside of your body. That's not a bad thing. In many ways, how you take care of the outside of your body has a lot of impact on how the rest of your body feels, including your happiness. That's why things like baths make you more relaxed and skin care can make you happier.

But self-care is a holistic experience, and it doesn't stop at just being good to your outsides. Think about it: You could spend a lot of time washing and detailing your car to keep it looking shiny and new, but if you never change the oil, it's never going to run properly. Your body is the same way. Focusing on what's going on inside can be hard because you don't see the effects as immediately as when you have a good hair day, for instance, but it's more about how it makes you feel and how healthy you are (in the long run).

Sleep is an obvious part of self-care (who among us doesn't love to be well-rested), but wellness as self-care involves more. Supplements can improve your mood, of course, and so can your sex life. These days you can also use things like cannabis to improve your bodily functions and cut pain (instead of just getting stoned). To really take your self-care to the next level, look at all areas of your life, not just your bathroom cabinet.

SUPPLEMENTS: MORE THAN JUST PROTEIN POWDER

Save for the daily multivitamin your mom made you take when you were a kid, when you think of a supplement, you probably think of protein powder. Most men do. Walk into any supplement store and the men's section is packed with swollen tubs of protein and aggressive pre-workout concoctions with names that sound like professional wrestlers. You'll also probably see a sprinkling of smaller jars promising better hair and better boners—sure, we want those too.

Supplements, however, aren't only about building muscle or having better sex. These days, new dietary supplements are designed for holistic health, which makes them perfect for self-care. For example, did you know that mushrooms can improve your mood, bacteria can help you lose weight, and certain proteins can help you get less wrinkly as you age? How's that for self-care?

Why Take Them?

The real question you should be asking is, "Why not take them?" Just like you turn to protein powder when you want to get swole, you can use dietary supplements to address a variety of other issues.

The problem is that unlike with protein powder, the effects are hard to measure. Think of it this way: If you take protein powder and work out, you'll probably see gains pretty quickly. But if you take a ground-up mushroom that helps you de-stress, those effects are harder to measure. It's more about a feeling than what you see in the mirror. But that doesn't mean they're not working.

Keep in mind as you read on, the most important thing about taking dietary supplements is consistency. Today's short attention spans expect quick results, but you have to take many of these consistently to see any difference. Even then, it may just be something you feel, so check in with your body every so often to see if you can feel any difference. Follow the directions on the package and don't think that taking more will bring you faster results. And like anything, ask your doctor if you have any questions or feel like you're getting negative side effects. Not all supplements will work for all people, and you should stop taking something if you don't like how it's making you feel.

Self-Care Supplements

The world of self-care supplements is vast and confusing. When you're browsing the aisles or cruising websites, look for some of these general categories to help guide you to the right place.

Probiotics

You might have heard people talking a lot recently about gut health and your body's microbiome. Basically, they're talking about thousands of bacteria that live on and inside your body and help it function properly. Lots of them live inside your gastrointestinal tract (they're called "gut flora") and help things, um, move along. Probiotic supplements help to keep these little guys around and can help control bloating, ease constipation, and more.

Prebiotics

Like with probiotics, taking a prebiotic supplement is all about optimizing your gut health. While probiotics are all about replacing gut flora that we may have lost, prebiotics are more about keeping them healthy. These supplements are usually talked about as food for the bacteria themselves and are used to make sure your existing gut flora is flourishing and healthy, and sticks around longer to do its job. When in doubt on which you need, look for a supplement that contains both.

Adaptogens

These supplements are like the celebrities of the wellness world—they're getting a lot of attention because of their ability to literally adapt to what your body needs. Most adaptogenic supplements will contain certain varieties of herbs or mushrooms, like ashwagandha, reishi, or lion's mane, which are popular in Eastern herbal medicine. They can do a lot of different things, thanks to their ability to reduce inflammation inside the body, but are most praised for their ability to naturally regulate your mood and decrease your stress.

Collagen

You may already know what collagen is: the part of your skin that keeps it tight and youthful looking. You may even be using an anti-aging serum that contains collagen. But topical applications can only take you so far. Collagen powders have been used in sports medicine for years to help alleviate joint pain and help patients recover from injuries and surgeries. In addition to helping your body heal, these powders can also keep your skin looking younger all over your body.

Omega-3

You've probably heard of people taking fish oil because of the omega-3s, and it actually does more than just make your burps taste like salmon. Omega-3s are essential building blocks to all types of cells found in your body, and while you probably won't see a lot of changes on the outside, they have been found to help with everything from heart disease to depression. They're definitely not sexy or trendy but are an important part of any wellness supplement routine.

Ginkgo Biloba

This ancient tree has been a cornerstone in Chinese herbal medicine for centuries and has recently become popular in wellness and self-care circles because of its ability to help increase the health and function of your brain. It comes down to its antioxidant and anti-inflammation properties, similar to those of an adaptogen, which can also help soothe muscle and joint pain. Taking ginkgo biloba and other brain-focused supplements could make you more alert without the aid of coffee in the morning and improve memory as well.

Biotin

An essential protein in the production of hair, biotin has been used as a topical hair loss treatment for years. Science is now supporting that taking biotin (and its cousin, keratin) orally could help build hair from the inside out. This is great news for men who are concerned with hair loss and thinning, specifically. New hair-focused supplements containing biotin claim they're more natural versions of the classic Propecia. Keep in mind that you'll need to take these supplements consistently for a minimum of three months to start seeing the effects.

Melatonin

Not all supplements are meant to take first thing in the morning. Melatonin, a natural sleep supporter, can help you get better quality sleep for longer without the aid of drugs like Ambien. Too many people don't get enough sleep on a regular basis, but using supplements can help. Some melatonin users have reported intense or strange dreams when using it, but the side effects are much less than with chemical sleep aids.

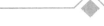

ARE ADAPTOGENS MAGIC?

Understanding how adaptogens work is confusing, even to medical professionals. In fact, no one truly knows how adaptogens do what they do, which is why they're often referred to as magic. What is known is that they have powerful antioxidant and anti-inflammatory properties. Many ailments in people's bodies are caused by inflammation, including everything from skin diseases to heart issues to some mood disorders. Adaptogens attack the root of a problem instead of the symptoms. "But I thought you said they reduce stress," you're saying. They do. When you're stressed your brain sends a signal to your body to enter fight-or-flight mode, which is meant to be a quick response. Consistent stress, however, makes your body stay in fight-or-flight mode, which causes sustained inflammation. Adaptogens won't calm you down immediately, but they will help manage stress in the long run.

EXERCISE FOR THE COUCH POTATO

Realistically, everyone knows exercise is good for them. Most people, however, think about working out as a way to look better (how else do you explain the popularity of "fitstagrammers"?). It's true: You can't have a sick body without putting work into it—though lord knows we've all tried.

Exercise, however, is one of the easiest things to integrate into a self-care routine, especially if you're already doing it. It's about changing your mentality. Instead of thinking about exercise in terms of how you look (or how it will make you look), start thinking about how it will make you feel. It's been shown that exercise has about a million other benefits apart from building a "beach body." Exercise shouldn't be a chore or something to check off your to-do list; it should be something that you want to do because it makes you feel good.

That might mean turning off *Instagram*, rethinking your gym, or finding a new class that you mesh with better. Being healthy isn't about how many squats you can do; it's about building a lifestyle and taking care of yourself.

Why You Should Exercise

If you're wondering why exercise is included in a book about self-care, it's because like anything that's good for you, it has a multitude of benefits. You'll notice, as well, that these benefits have nothing to do with how you look in a bathing suit. That's because self-care is about how well you're taking care of your body, not only for the aesthetic value. Sure, exercising regularly will make you look better, but even moderate exercise (20 minutes a day) can have a significant impact on your entire life. Here's how.

Controls Weight

Perhaps most obviously, even moderate exercise will help keep your body weight under control. It's basic physiology. If you eat more calories than you burn, you will gain weight; if you eat fewer, you will lose weight. But whether you are trying to lose weight or not, burning calories on a regular basis will help your body function better and store less fat.

Helps Prevent Heart Disease

File this under "everyone needs this." Heart disease kills about 340,000 men every year in the United States, according to the Centers for Disease Control and Prevention, and even moderate exercise can keep it at bay. Cardiovascular exercise, anything that raises your heart rate, will help strengthen your heart and lower your blood pressure, both of which are factors in your risk of heart disease.

Boosts Energy

Exercising releases hormones called endorphins in your brain, which are responsible for that energetic feeling you get after a workout. Exercising also helps your heart work better, which allows more oxygen to be pumped more effectively to other parts of your body. Experts say that the best cure for feeling sluggish isn't a cup of coffee; it's exercise.

Raises Your Mood

Those same endorphins that help boost your energy after a workout are also responsible for actually making you feel happier. These chemicals in your brain help to decrease pain and manage stress, and the more we exercise, the more endorphins we have. Remember that scene from *Legally Blonde* ("Exercise gives you endorphins. Endorphins make you happy. Happy people just don't kill their husbands.")? It's true.

Promotes Better Sleep

Expending energy during the day can have implications well into the night. Similar to how endorphins help raise your mood and alertness, even moderate exercise has been shown to help people fall asleep faster and stay asleep longer. Some have even said that having more muscle mass can improve your sleep, so don't discount the bicep curls either.

Leads to Better Sex

Most obviously, thinking you look better can give you more confidence in the sack. The sexual benefits of exercise extend to more than just what you see in the mirror (or what your partner is seeing during the act). That same increased blood flow that helps prevent heart disease can also help everything work better, particularly if you have erection issues.

Exercise for the Gym-Phobic

If you're not one of those guys who enjoys exercising, it can be hard to do it. The truth is, there is no right exercise for everyone, but any exercise is right for everyone. Taking care of yourself with exercise doesn't mean joining a fancy gym; it can be as simple as making some of these small changes.

Stretching

Stretching before exercise is always important to help prevent injury, but the stretching itself can be exercise if you do it right. It's often referred to as active or dynamic stretching and involves moving through the stretches instead of holding a static position. It will not only increase flexibility but also raise your heart rate. Here are some stretches to try:

To do a neck stretch, tilt your head toward your shoulder without twisting your neck. You should feel the neck pull on the opposite side. Do this once for 15 seconds. Repeat on the other side.

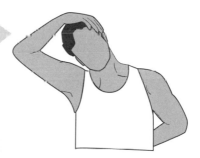

To try a lateral shoulder stretch, raise one arm overhead, grasp it with the other hand, and pull the elbow slowly behind the head. Hold this position for 15 seconds. Do once on each side.

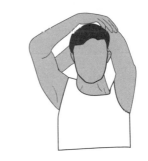

To do a posterior shoulder stretch, place your right hand on your left shoulder. Then, using your right hand, pull your left arm across the chest toward the right shoulder. Hold this position for 15 seconds. Repeat for the other shoulder.

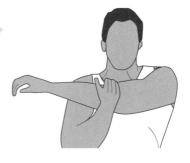

For a bridge stretch, lift your arms above your head, interlacing your fingers if possible, and straighten your elbows. Reach as high as possible. Hold for 15 seconds.

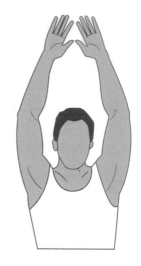

Here's a good stretch for your lower back: Stand with your feet shoulder-width apart. Then twist while leaning forward to touch your toes with the opposite hand. Extend your other arm up behind you. Hold for 5 seconds. Repeat on the opposite side.

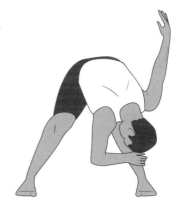

To do an inner-thigh stretch, stand with your feet shoulder-width apart and point your toes forward. Bend your right knee slightly and move your left hip downward toward the right knee. Hold for 15 seconds and repeat for the other leg.

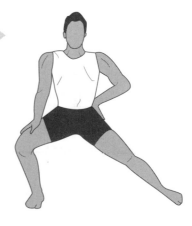

Walking

Thanks to wearable fitness devices, walking has never been cooler. They measure how many steps you take and keep you on track (they say you should be taking about 10,000 steps a day). They're great for reminding you to make small changes, like parking farther away from the entrance to a store or walking a few blocks instead of hopping on the bus.

Take the Stairs

Any time you come to an elevator, try to take the stairs instead, especially if it's just a few flights. The aerobic exercise of walking up stairs increases your heart rate exponentially and can help build muscle in your legs and butt. It's one of the simplest things you can do for the most benefit.

Body Weight Moves

You don't need to use fancy machines to exercise; body weight movements can be just as good. Most experts recommend a series of easy moves like push-ups, lunges, and squats to help raise your heart rate and build muscle without weights. The benefit is that these can be done anywhere: your bedroom, your hotel room, or even your office.

Ride a Bike

Bike riding has become all the rage in cities across the country, and it's a great way to get in exercise throughout the day. Instead of driving or taking public transportation, get a bike (or use one of the many bike-sharing services) and use that instead. You'll get aerobic exercise benefits as well as getting where you're going quicker than walking. Just, please, always wear a helmet.

Get an App

Thanks to modern technology, there are now all sorts of fitness apps that hold you accountable for exercise. Most apps include at-home exercise routines, many of which are body-weight-focused, and allow you to work out on the go or in the privacy of your home. You can even set alerts to remind you to work out if fitting exercise into your schedule is hard for you.

Yoga

Yoga, similar to active stretching, has the benefit of making you more flexible while also raising your heart rate. It's minimal impact, which means unlike things like running, it's also good for people with joint issues. Studies have shown that it can even help with insomnia.

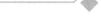

THE WORKOUT MONTAGE

Rocky Balboa running up the steps of the Philadelphia Museum of Art. The Karate Kid learning wax on, wax off. Luke Skywalker carrying Yoda on his back. Popular culture has perfected the art of the cinematic training montage. They're fun to watch, sure, but also can be misleading. They make hard work and the change that comes with it seem easy. How many times have you wished you could fast-forward to where you have a six-pack and can climb to the top of the rope? If it were as easy as in the movies, everyone would do it. Be careful of comparing yourself—everyone has their own journey. But workout montages do come in handy when you want to get motivated AF.

THE TRUTH ABOUT DETOXING

At the most basic level, detoxing or cleansing is designed to rid your body of toxins. These toxins don't have to be substances like drugs or alcohol even though we use the same terminology. Toxins could come from anywhere: pollution in your environment; chemicals, preservatives, or pesticides in your food; or a host of other places. The idea is that your body can build up reserves of all sorts of toxins that can affect how well you function. By detoxing, you're cleansing your system and flushing them out. Usually this involves fasting or sticking to a strict diet for a set period of time to allow your body to get rid of anything harmful.

Most detox programs target the liver, kidneys, and gut, which act as your body's filtration system and can get clogged with debris just like your shower drain. A detox cleanse can help flush out the bad stuff from these areas to help them filter more properly. Think of it as Drano for your body.

Why Do It?

Cleansing enthusiasts claim that by going through regular detoxes, their bodies are able to function at a higher level. Sometimes toxins can build up in people's bodies over time and they don't even realize that they're feeling bad. Maybe you have chronic headaches that you can't explain or you've been feeling sluggish for a few weeks. Maybe you find that it's harder to get through your regular workouts or you feel more bloated than usual. Maybe your allergies are a little bit worse lately. A detox cleanse, in theory, could help you feel better because you're essentially resetting your body. But your reason for doing a cleanse doesn't need to be so thought out. Maybe you partied a little too hard on vacation or drank too much at your friend's bachelor party and you just want to feel better—that's a good reason too.

What To Know Before You Start

Before you start any cleanse, you should consult your doctor. They'll be able to let you know if you have any health issues that you should keep in mind when cleansing. Keep in mind that not everyone is a fan of cleanses, so listen to what they have to say with an open mind. If you move forward with the cleanse, no matter what type, there are side effects. Be prepared to be irritable and moody at some point. You may also feel lethargic or even have flu-like symptoms the first few days. This is all part of your body going through withdrawal from things it might be used to (like sugar and carbs). The more decadent your lifestyle is before the cleanse, the harder the cleanse might be for you. Cleanses only work if you stick with them, so choose one that you think you can follow. For example, if you've never done one before, don't try to do a three-week juice cleanse right off the bat; start with a couple days to see how you like it.

Types of Detox Cleanses

All cleanses work on the same goal: eliminating the bad things from your diet. How you do that is up to you.

Juice Cleanse

These detoxes are the most popular and usually involve eliminating all solid food from your diet in favor of fresh juices. You'll typically drink five or six juices a day for anywhere from a few days to a few weeks depending on what kind you're doing. While you get lots of nourishment from the juices, they can be hard for some people who miss the sensation of chewing (some cleanses will let you eat certain low-calorie foods like celery to help with that).

Fasting

This is the OG detox cleanse where you literally eat nothing for a set amount of time. These days, you hear a lot about intermittent fasting, which is when you only eat for a set window each day (typically afternoon). Other fasting cleanses allow you to eat certain foods only at night. Theoretically, you are resetting your body to listen to itself more and use up stored nutrients instead of constantly eating new ones. The key, in all cases, is to drink a lot of water.

Elimination Diet

These diets ask you to eat a very restricted diet, usually only lean proteins and certain vegetables. They were once used to help figure out what foods someone was allergic to (after you reset your body, you gradually introduce certain food groups). These days, this diet is used in detoxing as well, especially if you're concerned about how your body reacts to things like gluten or sugar.

Colon Cleanse

Like the name suggests, this type of cleanse specifically targets the colon and GI tract and is meant to deal with issues like constipation, bloating, and irregularity. These cleanses come in all forms, from high-fiber shakes to just drinking salt water (which cannot be absorbed by the body). It's best when done under the supervision of a medical professional, since damage to your GI tract is a possibility and can lead to bigger issues down the road.

Liver Cleanse

This type of cleanse also targets a specific area of the body: the liver. Your liver helps filter out the bad stuff that comes into your body, flushes out waste, and helps process nutrients. Liver cleanses are especially attractive to people who drink a lot of alcohol or live an especially unhealthy lifestyle. Liver cleanses will often involve a restricted or juice diet and may also require additional supplements. Keep in mind, though, that the science is still out on whether these truly work or not.

Bone Broth Cleanse

Like fasting or a juice cleanse, this detox program restricts your diet for a set period of time. In this case, you only drink bone broth, which was made popular by the Paleo movement. These cleanses are short, usually lasting only a couple of days, and are thought to completely reset your body while still giving it some of the nutrients and protein it needs to function.

A NOTE ON POOPING

Point blank: Pooping can be an issue on a cleanse. That's because you may be drinking only juice or broth and those things do not have very much fiber. If you're fasting, then you're not eating anything at all, so not only is your fiber low but you don't have as much waste to get rid of. Some people get colonics while they're cleansing to help clean out what's stuck and keep things moving. Others just go with the (lack of) flow and hope for the best once the cleanse is over. Never try to force it; wait for it to happen naturally. Pro tip: When your cleanse is over, start with easy-to-digest foods that are high in fiber to make sure things are moving smoothly. Sometimes, on a juice cleanse, you might poop *more*. That's because it's doing what it's supposed to do and your body is getting rid of built-up waste and toxins. Either way, the goal is to get the toxins out, and honestly, is there a better way?

SLEEP: THE MOST IMPORTANT PART OF YOUR DAY

How many times have you said, "I'll sleep when I'm dead" in favor of partying, working, or choosing anything else over a healthy night's sleep? Sleep may seem trivial, especially when you're young, but it's an important bodily function. While you're sleeping, your body has the opportunity to repair itself, produce important hormones that support bodily functions and development, and even help your brain work better. And if you think sleep is for the weak, you have it backward.

Sleep deprivation can have both a physical and mental effect on you. When you don't get enough sleep, you have less energy and become, in fact, weaker. Your brain doesn't work as actively and you can develop memory issues. Long-term lack of sleep has even been linked to heart failure and strokes. Issues like insomnia and sleep apnea, when left untreated, can actually be life threatening.

You probably already know all of this on some level. After all, who hasn't felt the effects of sleep deprivation after a week of staying late at the office or a particularly party-heavy vacation. But building a healthy sleep routine and making sure your body has enough time to sleep is one of the most important parts of any self-care regimen. In truth, many of the tenets of self-care are meant to facilitate relaxation and, by extension, sleep. Sleeping when you're stressed is difficult, and self-care is one of the best ways to alleviate that stress. The first step is to change the way you think about sleep from something you have to do to something your body needs, and maybe eventually to something you want to do.

What Is Deep Sleep?

The human sleep cycle has four stages ranging from light sleep to deep sleep. Stage four is the deepest sleep where all the magic happens. Your body relaxes, your breathing slows, and your heart rate and body temperature lower. This is when your body does the most to heal itself—tissues are repaired, important hormones are made and released, and your brain is able to produce memories and process learning.

Studies have shown that as much as 23 percent of your sleep every night should be deep sleep (about 90 minutes a night). However, since you have to go through three stages of sleep to get there, it requires hours of quality sleep leading up to it. If you have sleep issues like insomnia or sleep apnea, it may not be possible to reach that phase at all. Without deep sleep, your body does not have the time it needs to rebuild, and the physical manifestations of this are sleep-deprivation symptoms like a foggy mind and fatigue.

How to Improve Your Sleep

For many people (maybe even you) sleep doesn't come easy. There are always so many other things we'd rather do; how many times have you said, "just one more episode?" But whether you're a good sleeper or a problem sleeper, building a constructive bedtime routine can make all the difference. It's called "sleep hygiene," and you should think about it the same way you do your daily shower.

Dim the Lights

It sounds obvious, but when there is too much light in your bedroom, it's harder to reach deep sleep. Make sure the light in the room is low and relaxing. If you get a lot of natural light during the day or live in a city where there is a lot of light pollution, you may want heavy blackout curtains to help block disruptive light. Some people find it easier to wake up in the morning with natural light, so if you're one of them, choose curtains or blinds that filter light instead of completely blocking it out.

Lower the Temperature

Make sure your room is cool, some studies have suggested as cool as 60°F. When you reach deep sleep, your body temperature actually lowers, and it's thought that a cooler room will help make it easier for your body to get there.

Get Rid of Screens

It's hard in today's world where you have a computer in your hand and TVs in every room in the house. The blue light from these screens, however, overstimulates your eyes and brain and makes relaxing harder. Experts say to turn off all screens at least an hour before bedtime. This could mean charging your phone in another room of the house or removing your TV from your bedroom.

Avoid Stimulants

Caffeine has such a stimulating effect that it can be felt even hours after your last cup of coffee. How sensitive you are to caffeine is personal, but most experts say to stop drinking caffeinated beverages like coffee, tea, or soda in the afternoon to make sure it's left your body by bedtime.

Start Your Routine Earlier

To help signal to your body and brain that it's time to sleep, develop a bedtime routine that you can start early. This may mean brushing your teeth or washing your face earlier or taking a relaxing bath with essential oils. It could also mean starting a meditation practice or doing some stretching. Whatever you choose to do, start it at least an hour before you get into bed and don't rush through it.

Don't Eat Too Late

Some experts say to not eat dinner after 8 p.m. because it hinders digestion. There is some truth there when it comes to sleep too, since active digestion takes energy. Eating too close to bedtime has also been said to lead to acid reflux and GI tract issues. Eating before 8 p.m. is a good benchmark, but it really depends on what time you're going to bed. Choose a time that works for your lifestyle, and make sure it's at least 2 hours before bedtime.

Get Good Sheets

Studies have shown that the type of sheets you sleep on matters to how quickly your body is able to reach deep sleep. It's important that your sheets help your body temperature stay low and don't trap heat. Some studies have shown that linen sheets actually help keep your body several degrees cooler than other materials like cotton. Cotton is a good standard for most people however. If you have sensitive skin, wash your sheets in an unscented detergent to prevent irritation that could keep you up at night.

Use a Noise Machine

Noise pollution, particularly if you live in a city, can be one of the biggest obstacles to getting enough sleep. If your bedroom is particularly noisy, you can use earplugs at night to block out noise or purchase a white noise machine to cover them up.

THE WATER QUESTION

Nighttime cramps, often in one's legs, are so common that some studies show that as many as 60 percent of adults get them regularly. While the reason behind them is not fully understood, one of the factors could be dehydration. Staying well hydrated throughout the day can show an improvement. But drinking a huge glass of water right before bedtime might not be the solution, particularly if you have an issue with getting up to use the bathroom in the middle of the night. It's a no-win scenario: You wake up because of a leg cramp or you wake up to pee, both of which will disrupt your sleep cycle. One solution could be to just drink more water throughout the day. The other could be a homeopathic remedy: drinking a shot of pickle brine before bed. The theory is that the salt in the brine will help you retain water throughout the night and keep your limbs hydrated.

HOW TO CHILL WITH CBD

Right around the time certain states started to legalize recreational marijuana use, you probably started hearing about CBD. It's popping up in everything from moisturizers to seltzer water; you can get CBD lattes at your coffee shop and CBD manicures at the local nail salon. And while eleven states have already legalized recreational weed, and more seem to be on the horizon, you don't have to live in one of them to be able to use CBD, because it won't get you high.

Unsurprisingly, the wellness community is full of early adopters of both weed and CBD, not to mention hemp. But as all these things become increasingly mainstream, they're met with even more confusion. The cultural obsession with feeling better and growing interest in self-care have birthed a whole new industry built on the pot leaf. In this section, the focus is going to stay on CBD because not only is it legal everywhere, it's also the most confusing to people. The bottom line is that CBD can take your self-care game to another level—as long as you know what it is and how to use it.

What Is CBD?

First things first: CBD will not get you stoned, so if you were expecting to chew a CBD gummy and drift off into a haze, you're going to be sadly disappointed. CBD is an abbreviation for a chemical called cannabidiol, which is a type of cannabinoid (of which there are thousands). Cannabinoids are chemicals derived from the cannabis (hemp) plant. THC, the chemical in weed that actually will get you high, is also a cannabinoid. This is where the confusion lies. THC and CBD are like your sister and brother: part of the same family, but inherently different. Even though there are thousands of different cannabinoids, the reason you hear the most about THC and CBD is that they are the ones that have been studied the most.

How Does It Work?

Science has recently discovered that the human body contains something called the endocannabinoid system, a complex system—closely linked to the endocrine and nervous systems—whose receptors specifically react to cannabinoids. When you come in contact with THC, for instance, it's the endocannabinoid system that gets you high (or that at least facilitates the process). The same goes for CBD, though it tells these receptors to send different signals.

In the case of CBD, it has been found to be a powerful anti-inflammatory agent and can help your body regulate pain. Many of your bodily ailments are caused by inflammation, including joint and muscle pain, so treating the root of the problem will treat the symptoms. As a result, CBD has been and is currently being studied to treat everything from digestion issues, chronic pain, and seizures to insomnia. In skin care, thanks to CBD's ability to work topically as well as orally, it's being looked at for acne, eczema, and anti-aging.

Why Is It in Everything?

The short answer is because everyone is crazy for it, so companies are rushing to come out with CBD products to capitalize on their obsession. The long answer, though, is that we haven't even begun to scratch the surface of its practical applications. Anecdotally, it's been used by enthusiasts "for years" to treat all sorts of ailments. Scientifically, we are only beginning to understand its capabilities. Basically, we're throwing everything at the wall to see what sticks.

Will It Work?

Like all things, you don't know if a CBD product is going to work until you try it. But there are a few indications that can help you cut through the CBD BS.

When you're looking at ingestible products like tinctures or gummies, look to see if they list the amount of CBD inside. It's usually in the form of milligrams, and the package will note how much is in the entire thing. Look at the usage instructions on the package; these usually list the amount per serving. This doesn't always mean that the more CBD there is, the better it will work, but if you've never used it before, start with a lower dose.

Whatever product you're using, look to see where CBD falls on the ingredients list. A general rule is the higher up on the list, the more of that ingredient is included in the formula. This means that if the list is long and CBD falls in the second half of it, there is very little in there and you probably won't get much benefit.

If you're using CBD in skin care, look to see what other ingredients are in the product. The biggest benefit of CBD is as an anti-inflammatory ingredient, so it's particularly good when paired with things like retinol or vitamin C, which can sometimes cause irritation. It can also be good in a soothing oil or cream to help calm redness and rosacea quicker.

How to Use CBD for Self-Care

Generally, how you use CBD depends on two things: what your desired results are and what product you've chosen to use. These are some of the most common:

Stress
CBD has been shown to help decrease stress immediately and help people manage it in the long run. Ingestible CBD is best for this, so look for tinctures, edible oils, and gummies. Its effects can compound over time, so look for something with a low dose designed to be used daily and take it like a vitamin.

Pain
One of the most common uses for CBD is to alleviate joint and muscle pain (and there is more science to back up this claim than most of the other uses). Look for balms and creams with a high percentage of CBD and apply them directly on the area that's hurting. Balms tend to have a bit more CBD in them while creams sometimes will have additional soothing ingredients like menthol.

Sleep
Thanks to CBD's calming influence on the body, it's commonly used as a natural sleep aid. These products are often taken orally and can come in the form of liquids or pills. Some have said that it's especially good when paired with melatonin when your focus is on sleep.

Skin
Topically, CBD is especially good when treating irritation like chronic eczema, rosacea, and sometimes even acne. If you have dry skin, look for products like oils or creams. For acne, look for

lighter-weight serums or gels. Most CBD skincare products are oil-based (since CBD is more stable when bound in an oil), so keep that in mind if acne or oily skin are problems for you.

CBD IS NOT HEMP OIL

Marketers would like you to be confused about CBD, because if you are, you might buy a product with hemp oil instead. But don't let the pot leaf on your moisturizer fool you. Hemp and CBD, while both derived from the same kind of plant, are very different. Hemp oil is extracted from the seed of a hemp plant and contains no cannabinoids. CBD, on the other hand, is derived from the entire plant itself. Hemp oil isn't bad; it contains a high amount of fatty acids and antioxidants that are good for you, especially your skin. But if you were hoping to get CBD-like effects from just run-of-the-mill hemp, you'll be disappointed.

SEX: WITH YOURSELF (AND OTHERS!)

Let's just put it out there: Everyone does it. Without sounding too Pollyanna about it all, masturbation is a fact of life. How often you do it, how you do it, or what you think about while you do it isn't important; it's the fact that you do it that makes you a human dude. Everyone has opinions on the rights and wrongs of jerking off from the *right* way to do it to whether doing it at all is *wrong*.

The goal of this section isn't to get into a discussion on whether it's okay to do it. The assumption is that you do, but you may not think of it as an act of self-care. For many men, masturbating is a means to an end. It's a way to alleviate anxiety or stress or pent-up sexual tension, something to be done when you're alone in the house, while you're watching dirty movies, or maybe to "clean the pipes" before getting busy with another human. But like most things that fall under the umbrella of self-care, it's not about what you're doing, it's about *why* you're doing it.

Masturbating has actual proven health benefits. Some say it can help lower the risk of prostate cancer. Others say it can improve your mood and your immune system. It has also been said to improve your heart health, help you sleep better, and even make your skin better. But one of the most important benefits can be harder to measure: Jerking off is self-care.

Wait, How Can Jerking Off Be Self-Care?

The way masturbation can improve your mood is similar to exercise. When you work out, you release endorphins, which help decrease stress and elevate your happiness. Orgasms also release hormones called dopamine and oxytocin, which make you happier as well as activate the pleasure sensors in your nervous system. This goes for any orgasm, whether you're having one with a partner or not.

But the self-care benefits of masturbation go beyond the physiological. Masturbating can help you get to know your body and form a positive relationship with it. It can help you become in tune with how your body responds to certain things. It can deepen the understanding you have of your body.

How Masturbating Improves Your Sex Life

A healthy solo sex routine can make sex with a partner better too. Some studies have shown that regular masturbation helps men with erectile issues stay harder by increasing blood flow to their groin area. Others have found that masturbation allows some men to last longer during sex, particularly if it's done an hour or so before the act (seems like *There's Something about Mary* was on to something).

As established, masturbation can improve your relationship with your own body, and when you have a good relationship with your body, a few things can happen. You can be less self-conscious with another person. It can also help you become more in tune with your desires and what brings you pleasure. Once you know what you like, you can ask your partner for it.

Some partners view masturbation as a sign that their partner is unsatisfied. The reality is that that's rarely the case. If your partner is not a fan of your solo sex practices, invite them to try mutual masturbation to show them that sex with yourself doesn't mean you don't want to have sex with them too. It's all part of the same picture.

How to Practice Mindful Masturbation

To make masturbation part of your self-care routine, the first thing to do is reframe your thinking. Instead of thinking of jerking off as something to do quickly and "get through," give yourself time to savor the experience. Check in with your body while you're doing it, and make it something you look forward to. Wellness folk are calling it "mindful masturbation," and it's a real thing. Here's how to do it.

Switch It Up

If you've always masturbated the same way, maybe even since you were a kid, you're missing the possibility of new experience. It could be as simple as switching your position (lie down if you usually stand up) or location (do it in the shower if you're usually in bed). It could also mean keeping quiet if you usually make a lot of noise or vice versa. Try to do something different each time to find out how your body responds.

Turn Off the Porn

Lots of men use porn to facilitate masturbation, and that's totally fine, but the problem comes from depending on it to get in the mood. If you usually watch porn when you masturbate, next time turn it off. Use your imagination instead. Think of previous sexual encounters or fantasize about new ones.

Touch Other Parts of Your Body

If you're masturbating with a goal in mind (i.e., an orgasm), you may rush through it and only focus on your hardware. Instead, take time to savor the experience and allow your hands to touch other parts of your body. Understand the sexual sensations of other parts of your body. It could be as simple as using a different hand, touching your nipples, stroking your inner thigh, or massaging your prostate area; all could lead to new, and better, sensations.

Try Edging

Instead of trying to come as quickly as possible, try to keep the orgasm at bay. In sexual circles, this is called edging, where you get yourself close to orgasm but don't finish the job. Get yourself to the edge of orgasm and then take a break. Once you've calmed down, start up again. Do this a few times in a row until you can't wait anymore. The result is a deeper orgasm.

Use Some Tools

Just like exploring other parts of your body, using different tools apart from your hands can open you up to new experiences you never had before (and never knew you liked). Try a masturbation sleeve, which is a toy meant to mimic the feeling of partner sex. Or consider a prostate stimulating tool or butt plug, which helps to massage the G-spot around your prostate and many say produces more full-body orgasms.

Can You Masturbate Too Much?

Remember that old wives' tale that if you masturbate too much you'll grow hair on your palms? That's not going to happen. The fact is that there is no set standard for what is "too much." How much you masturbate is personal, and while there aren't any specific health conditions that stem from excessive masturbation, there are a few warning signs that you should ease up. If you physically hurt yourself masturbating, like are rubbing your penis so much that the skin becomes irritated or chafed, then you need to take a break. If you're masturbating so much that it's interfering with your ability to do your job or keep relationships, that's an issue. And if you are preoccupied with the thought or act of masturbation, then that could be the sign of a compulsion.

AS AMERICAN AS APPLE PIE

When *American Pie* hit theaters in 1999, on the surface it was just the next in a long line of raunchy, teenage sex romp movies. But the iconic scene, where the main character Jim Levenstein masturbates with an apple pie, isn't just the movie's namesake. The scene is funny, of course, but also promotes the idea that masturbation, and experimentation with masturbation, is normal. Did many young dudes run out and buy baked goods to use as Fleshlights after seeing the movie? Probably not. But it was one of the first times in mainstream media that masturbation wasn't portrayed as something shameful or quick. Masturbation should be experimental and fun—there's no shame in that.

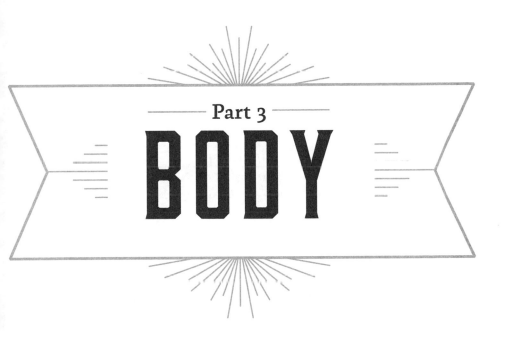

Part 3

BODY

When you think about taking care of your body, you tend to focus on what's going on inside. That, of course, is important, but what you might not consider is how taking care of the outside of your body affects your well-being too.

General hygiene is more than just something you do because you have to. It can have a real impact on your long-term health. But there is so much more to it than that. What you do for your body has a real impact on your mental health and mood. Aromatherapy, for instance, is based on the idea that certain smells can alter your brain chemistry and facilitate relaxation and sleep or have an energizing effect. Aromatherapy, for that reason, is a common component of things like baths, massages, and even personal use products like lotions and oils.

Self-care for your body isn't just focused on relaxation. Tattoos can be a form of self-care, because they are something you're consciously doing to create the body you want. That desire is at the core of self-care: doing something because it helps create the person you want to be. So whatever your goals are, whether you want to transform your outward appearance or just not stink, taking care of your body properly can be one of the most helpful things you can do.

SKIP THE SHOWER. YOU SHOULD BE TAKING BATHS.

You probably haven't taken a bath since you were a little kid, and there's a reason for that. Baths are a commitment. Showers are functional and (can be) quick, but baths mean literally clearing your schedule for what can seem like an unnecessary amount of time. Not to mention, in increasingly screen-obsessed lives, purposefully doing something that prohibits the use of screens seems like self-torture.

Those two things are precisely why baths have become a cornerstone of the self-care movement. They force you to take time out of your life and do something by yourself (unless you're using a bath for, you know, sexy reasons). Baths are solitary; they force you to be alone with your thoughts without the benefit of distraction. Baths are also relaxing as hell, which is why when you think of a bath, you probably think of one of those *Instagram* pics of a bath full of rose petals and surrounded by so many candles it looks like a vigil. It's true, some people really go all out with their baths, but you don't have to go through an entire book of matches and an Enya album to reap the benefits.

The benefits? They're plentiful and go well beyond getting clean. Has anyone ever told you, "To get really clean, take a bath"?

That's true: Nothing will get you as clean as being submerged in water for a long period of time. When we start talking about baths for self-care, though, the reasoning goes well beyond just giving yourself a good scrub down. Baths can actually make real changes in your mood, internal bodily functions, and long-term health.

The Health Benefits of Baths

Bathing has been the cornerstone to wellness in many cultures for centuries. The Japanese even have a name for bathing for wellness: *onsen*. What they know that you don't is that bathing can heal a variety of ailments, and science is starting to back them up.

Improve Your Mood

Some studies have shown that submerging your body in water unlocks feelings of being in a womb, which in turn bring feelings of comfort and security. These same studies have shown that bathing can quell anxiety and decrease depression and feelings of pessimism.

Muscle Recovery

The reason you'll often find bathtubs in sports medicine offices? Hot baths increase circulation, which can help ease muscle pain and soften tight muscles. On the flip side, ice-cold baths restrict the blood vessels and can help reduce swelling and speed up muscle regeneration.

Better Sleep

It's been found that when you sleep your body temperature drops, which helps produce melatonin, a natural substance that helps you sleep. Many say that taking a hot bath before bed helps facilitate this process by raising your body temperature and making this internal temperature change happen quicker.

Strengthen Your Immune System

Not only will the steam from a hot bath help ease congestion but the warm water itself could help fight off disease in the first place. Studies have shown that certain cells in your immune system may work more effectively at higher temperatures, which a bath can help induce.

Help Your Heart

Some studies have shown that regular hot baths can be effective at reducing blood pressure. The heat of the water increases blood flow and circulation, and lower blood pressure has been shown to decrease the likelihood of heart attack and stroke.

Burn Calories

Other studies have shown that this same ability to increase blood flow has a cardiovascular effect similar to exercise. Hot baths can raise your heart rate and cause you to sweat in a way similar to aerobic exercise (one study even found that an hour-long hot bath may burn as many calories as a brisk walk).

Soothe Skin

Warm baths, accompanied with essential oils and other soothing ingredients, have been shown to reduce inflammation in the skin, which is what's behind eczema, psoriasis, and even sunburn. They can even help standard dry skin by hydrating your body more completely than just applying creams and lotions (though very hot baths have been said to have the opposite effect and can be very drying).

Ease Arthritis Pain

The same muscle-loosening aspects of a hot bath can also have an effect on loosening stiff joints. Adding Epsom salt, which many say is easily absorbed into the skin through hot water, can help with pain management and further help to lubricate stiff joints.

Making the Perfect Bath

Now that you know the benefits of a bath it's time to start creating one. Here are the ingredients for a good bath:

- **Water:** It goes without saying. Just make sure it's not too hot since that can cause burns.
- **Salt:** Salt, especially Epsom salt, can help ease muscles, promote mineral absorption, and facilitate relaxation.
- **Essential oils:** Not only do certain essential oils have different properties when absorbed through the skin, like to promote sleep or healing, the scents provide additional aromatherapy.
- **Oatmeal:** The kind of oatmeal typically found in bathing products is colloidal oatmeal, which means it's been ground and suspended in liquid, and is particularly good at soothing skin ailments.
- **Baking soda:** Even the kind found in your kitchen cabinet can act as a powerful exfoliator and help remove calluses and dead skin.
- **Ice cubes:** Ice-cold baths aren't as relaxing but can be beneficial in muscle recovery and post-workout healing.

THINGS TO DO IN THE BATH

Because you have some time to kill, you could:

- **Read:** An actual book, not your iPad.
- **Think:** When else are you going to decompress from your day?
- **Meditate:** It's the perfect time to clear your mind.
- **Clean your fingernails:** Seriously, you need to.
- **Listen to music:** Just make sure the speaker is far away from the water.

WHAT I DO: TOM FORD

Fashion designer Tom Ford is tasteful to the point of fastidiousness. His entire life (home, wardrobe, smells) is so put together it seems fake. Case in point, when explaining his daily routine to *Harper's Bazaar* in 2012, he admitted to taking four baths a day. "I lie in the tub for half an hour and just let my mind wander. I find a bath meditative," he said. By normal guy standards, multiple baths a day seems excessive, but Ford is definitely on to something. Baths can be restorative and they can also be energizing. It depends on what you do and what you need out of it. Still, so many baths a day is unrealistic, even for Ford. In another interview in 2015, he admitted his bathing had decreased to just one bath a day after becoming a father.

EVERY MAN NEEDS A MANICURE... AND A PEDICURE

One reason to take care of your hands and feet: Your partner really wants you to. Overwhelmingly, women say clean nails and smooth feet are things they find attractive in a man. After all, who really wants to feel like they're being rubbed with sandpaper when they're about to get busy?

For some men, this reason alone is enough to consider getting manicures and pedicures, but really, you should be getting them for *yourself*. We are talking about self-care after all, and the keyword is "self." This is a judgment-free zone, so whatever your reason is for considering nail, hand, and foot maintenance, run with it. Chances are, once you start doing it, you'll end up enjoying it yourself.

The bottom line is this: Every human being, male or female, needs to take care of their appendages. Hands are the workhorses of the body; they are the most-used tools in people's lives. Feet are the unsung heroes of your body; you might not think about them much, but they do the most. When either of these things is uncomfortable or, worse, in pain, it can have a serious impact on your life.

If your hands are routinely exposed to the world (like, if you don't wear gloves all day every day), you need to take care of them. If you work with your hands or depend on them for your livelihood, you definitely need to take care of them. If you wear sandals ever, you need to take care of your feet. If you are ever barefoot in public (like a gym locker room) or even just at home, you most certainly need to know what's going on with them and take steps to make sure they're clean and healthy.

Manicures and pedicures aren't just for aesthetics. They help keep your most-used appendages clean and healthy. They also feel freaking amazing. As self-care devices, manicures and pedicures take very little effort and deliver big results. Sure, you could clip your nails at home, but getting a professional manicure is next level; it's next to impossible to get your hands to feel the way a pro can no matter how much hand cream you slather on. Pedicures are even more incredible; there is a specific pleasure to having another person massage, exfoliate, and moisturize your feet.

Professional manicures and pedicures are low-cost and low-risk but do wonders for your mood (not to mention your hygiene). Depending on how fast your nails grow, you can get them as often as you want (even as often as once a week). But they're certainly not required for an effective self-care experience. You can do them yourself too. The most important thing is that you're doing it.

Why Get a Manicure?

Keeping your fingernails trimmed and clean can do wonders for your appearance, but there are actual health reasons for getting a manicure. Regularly trimming and cleaning fingernails can help keep them strong and prevent them from getting brittle or becoming ingrown. It can also prevent bacteria and fungus from growing and causing long-term finger and nail issues. Regularly moisturizing cuticles can prevent hangnails and help facilitate nail growth as well. Furthermore, most professional manicures come with a hand massage, which helps stimulate blood flow as well as relax your entire body (thanks to the series of pressure points in your hands). Some will also offer exfoliation, which helps to get rid of dead skin and prevent calluses from building.

What's a Pedicure?

Pedicures follow the same general procedure as a manicure, except on your feet. For men who tend to neglect their feet even more than their hands, they can be even more important. Your feet are hothouses of bacteria, especially if you routinely walk barefoot on tile floors or wear sandals. And since you probably keep them in shoes much of the time, bacteria and fungus, which flourish in moist, dark environments, can thrive. Ingrown toenails can increase the risk of bacterial infections, which can be painful. Athlete's foot, a fungus, can be itchy and painful if left untreated. It's even possible for your feet to develop dangerous skin cancers like melanoma and basal cell carcinoma (Bob Marley died from an unchecked melanoma on his foot, after all). Getting a pedicure won't cure cancer, but it could mean early detection.

Steps of a Manicure/Pedicure

Most manicures and pedicures follow the same formula. Here's what to expect no matter where you go, nail polish not required.

Clean
The technician will clean the surface of your nails to get rid of dirt and, depending on the length, will clean underneath them as well.

Cut

Then they'll cut your nails with a nail clipper based on how long you want them and what shape (usually rounded).

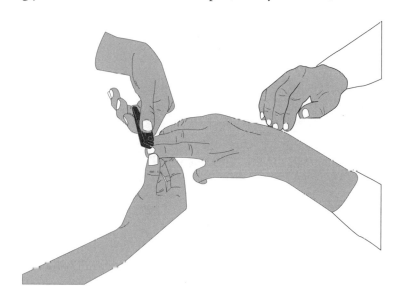

File

After the nails are cut, the technician will use a nail file to smooth the ends and make sure they're even and not rough.

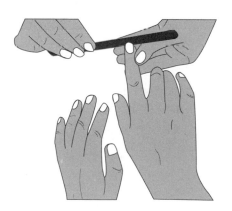

Soak

Usually you'll be asked to dip your fingertips in a bowl of liquid in order to moisturize the nails and cuticles. Afterward, they may apply a cuticle oil for further hydration.

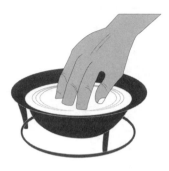

Push

Pushing is when the technician uses a tool to gently "push" the cuticle skin off the surface of the fingernail to make trimming it easier. This is optional, but if you have a problem with hangnails it can be beneficial.

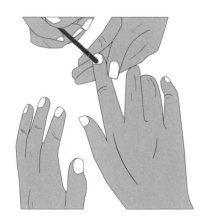

Moisturize

Depending on what you need, the technician may apply a scrub to exfoliate your hands before applying moisturizing cream. The cream application is usually done with a relaxing hand massage.

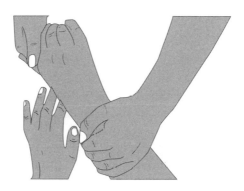

Buff

If you don't want polish, you have the option of getting your nails buffed, which leaves them shiny and healthy looking. Or you could opt for polish: clear or colored, whatever floats your boat.

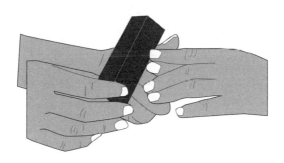

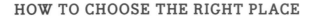

HOW TO CHOOSE THE RIGHT PLACE

The biggest risk of a pedicure is cross-contamination, so make sure you see the technician open a new package of tools in front of you before clipping and cutting. You should be able to clearly see the licenses of the person working on you. Since pedicures require putting your feet into a soaking basin, make sure you're not putting your feet into an already-filled bath and that there is a plastic liner. Checking online review sites is always a good way to get an idea of what type of experience you'll have. If you walk in and see another man there, that's a good sign too.

HOW TO DO A DIY PEDICURE

If getting a pedicure in public isn't your thing, here's how to do one in the comfort of your own home.

1. Soak your feet in a bath of warm water and Epsom salt for about 10 minutes. The soak helps soften your skin and calluses for easier exfoliation.
2. While still in the soak, use a foot scrub to exfoliate dead skin and get rid of calluses and a pumice stone to smooth away calluses.
3. Clip your toenails with a straight-edge clipper. Be careful to not cut them too short, which can be painful and invite fungus.
4. File the edges of your nails with a nail file or emery board to keep them smooth.
5. Apply a moisturizing foot cream all over your feet and even between your toes, and make sure you rub it in completely.

LOTION: IT DOESN'T HAVE TO BE GROSS

Proper skin care is important in your self-care practice to keep you looking great and also help protect your skin from issues down the road (more on this in Part 4). Well, the same philosophy goes into taking care of the skin on your body. There are subtle differences between facial skin and body skin (thickness, oil production, and hair follicles among them), but the general tenets of skin care still apply.

Still, like on their faces, most men are not taught to care for their bodies the way women are. This lack of knowledge leaves their skin particularly vulnerable to aging and other skin issues caused by inflammation and dehydration. Unless you already have an issue with dry skin, chances are you're not paying attention to the skin below your neck.

This is mostly because lotion is gross. At least, it can be. The way most men think of lotion is akin to sunscreen: a goopy, messy product that leaves you feeling greasy and uncomfortable. Men would rather forgo lotion completely and deal with the repercussions later than have to walk around with a film over their entire bodies, making it awkward and uncomfortable to move. Not to mention, many lotions smell terrible.

Men see lotion and other forms of body moisturizing as a tool to fix something (like chapped hands or crusty elbows) instead of something to prevent those things in the first place. In fact, we're taught from an early age that a soft hand isn't manly and rough patches are signs of ruggedness. In reality, self-care doesn't take away from your masculinity and neither does using lotion. In fact, it takes a confident and strong man to know what his body needs to be healthy and actually do it, soft hands be damned.

Taking care of your body in a meaningful way isn't hard. It's as easy as switching your body wash and finding a lotion you can actually stomach using (seriously, they're out there). The most important thing in consistency. Too many men use things like lotion only when they think they need it, and at that point, it takes a really long time to work. After all, once your hands are so cracked from winter wind that they're bleeding, lotion can only take you so far. Once you find a lotion or body oil that you actually like, start using it regularly, as often as you can remember. It's one of the easiest self-care moves you can make.

Why Skin Care for Your Body Is Important

Taking your skincare routine downtown, like to your torso, arms, hands, and yes, even lower, is important for the same reasons you take care of your face. Things like exfoliation and hydration can not only improve the immediate look of your skin, particularly if you have tattoos (we'll get to those later), but also ensure that the skin cells on your body are working the best they can. In order to do this, they need to be turned over (exfoliation), hydrated (moisturizing), and kept clean (washing).

Men are also prone to inflammatory skin issues on their bodies, like eczema and psoriasis, which are characterized by chronic dryness, itchiness, flaking, and irritation. Not taking care of your skin properly makes these issues worse, and using things like lotions and proper cleansers can help keep them at bay. If eczema and psoriasis are issues for you, seek the advice of a doctor to find out how best to manage them (gentle, unscented lotion is only the beginning). Even for men who don't struggle with these issues but do get dry skin occasionally from things like outdoor sports, taking care of the skin on your body is an important part in dealing with it.

What to Do

The good news is that an effective skincare routine for your body doesn't require a ton of steps.

Cleanse

The type of cleanser you use on your body is important. Make sure you're using a gentle cleanser that doesn't strip your skin completely (that telltale squeaky-clean feeling is not good). Instead, look for cleansers and body washes with moisturizing ingredients designed for sensitive skin. If you're especially sweaty, you may want to consider one of the many options with charcoal, which helps absorb dirt easily. Lots of men's body washes contain ingredients like tea tree and peppermint oil, but those can be irritating and drying if you have sensitive skin.

Exfoliate

The skin on your body has a life cycle about twenty-eight days long. Dead skin cells can accumulate on the surface and need to be cleared to make way for the smoother, better-looking skin beneath. For some people, a loofah sponge can do the trick. Also, consider using a body scrub or exfoliating wash with salicylic acid every so often, especially if you're prone to body acne (which is actually folliculitis, an inflammation of hair follicles, and can be avoided by regular exfoliation).

Lotion

After showering, apply a moisturizing lotion. The lotion will not only help lock in the moisture still on your skin from the shower, but will also have additional moisturizing ingredients to help keep skin hydrated. Look for lightweight formulas that won't leave you feeling sticky or filmy. Use a fragrance-free lotion if you're sensitive to fragrance or have irritation-prone skin. Lotions are best suited for people with especially dry skin and anyone with chronic issues like eczema.

Oil

If lotions aren't your thing, try a body oil instead. These oils typically use natural ingredients and essential oils to help hydrate skin and keep it moisturized just like a lotion, but can feel more lightweight and dry faster. They're also best when used directly out of the shower. The main difference between oils and lotions though is that lotions have ingredients called humectants, which actually draw moisture from the air and put it into your skin, while oils don't. Oils will soften skin by retaining moisture but won't actually moisturize skin on their own.

WTF IS CHAFING?

There is not a man in the world who hasn't dealt with chafing. Any time unprotected skin rubs together, like under your arms, between your butt cheeks, or on your inner thighs, the skin can get dry and irritated. It happens especially when you're active and skin rubs together quicker and longer. In the best cases, chafing is uncomfortable; in the worst, it can cause lesions that can get infected. The best way to prevent chafing is to use a lotion containing zinc oxide on the area regularly (it creates a protective barrier on top of skin). There are also special chafing products like sticks and lotions that use powders and other ingredients to create more "slip" so skin doesn't rub together.

TAN THE MAN

Being tan is a status symbol. It means you've spent time outside instead of locked away in a cubicle. It also implies that you're healthy since pale complexions are subconsciously associated with sickness. This is especially true for men since we as a culture still value male ruggedness. Men who spend all their time inside are sometimes thought to be less desirable than those who are perceived as active and vital.

Whether or not you think about these things often, you probably think you look better with a tan. Color in your skin has the ability to hide imperfections, smooth the appearance of skin, and even mask the appearance of blemishes like real-life Photoshop. It can also be an optical illusion by highlighting muscle tone (that's why bodybuilders are always very, *very* tan).

But we're in a tough spot. We still want to be tan, as a culture, but we also know that getting tan the traditional way is very bad. The science behind the effects of UV rays (sun damage, premature aging, skin cancer) is enough to keep you locked in your house with the shades drawn. How do you justify your deep need to be tan with your knowledge that it could kill you? There are plenty of ways.

How You Get Tan

To understand why tanning can be risky, you first need to understand how you get tan in the first place. It's all thanks to UV rays from the sun, which penetrate the top layer of your skin. There they trigger the production of melanin, the substance that produces dark pigment and keeps your skin from burning and is what gives people different skin tones. As melanin is produced, your skin gradually gets darker. Your body has a limit to how much melanin it can produce and once that limit has been reached, sunburn happens (regardless of how much sunscreen you're wearing).

Why Is It Bad?

The production of melanin isn't bad, but pushing the limit is. Once your body's natural defenses are spent, the UV rays begin to damage the very DNA of your cells. Your body floods the areas with blood to try to help heal the damaged cells. This can mean a painful, inflamed sunburn in the short term and mutated cells that lead to skin cancer in the long term.

UV rays also create free radicals, tiny molecules that steal electrons from others and damage them in the process. Free radical damage has also been linked to skin cancer as well as premature aging. The issue with all of this is that sun damage from UV rays is unavoidable but can be controlled; purposefully damaging the skin in order to obtain a golden tan is walking a dangerous line.

What to Do to Get a Tan (Safely)

Despite the negative effects of UV rays on your long-term health, you probably don't want to spend your life as pale as a ghost. After all, this knowledge hasn't done a lot to change your obsession with being tan. Luckily, along with this knowledge comes ways to get tan safer and quicker than frying on a beach.

Wear Sunscreen

Sunscreen is your best defense against the sun's damaging rays (see Part 4 for more on this). You should be wearing it every day, especially on your face. It's even more important any time you're purposefully spending long periods of time outside. You'll still get tan, but it may just take longer. Remember to never use sunscreen with less than SPF 30.

Sunless Tanning

Sunless tanning products use a chemical called dihydroxyacetone (DHA), which reacts to dead cells on the surface of your skin and temporarily darkens them. It's not the same melanin-producing process as getting a natural tan and doesn't last quite as long, but gives the look of a tan without risking skin cancer down the road. Sunless tanning products come in a variety of forms like sprays, mousses, creams, and drops. Most of them give only slight color in one use and are designed to use consistently until you build up the color you want. At-home products are plentiful, but professional spray tans are also available and exceedingly popular for the same reason you don't want to cut your own hair: They look far better if left to a professional.

Bronzer

Bronzers are useful for a very temporary tan fix, especially on your face. They come in a variety of forms like powder, gels, and creams and are useful if you want to look tan immediately. The easiest bronzers for most men to use are gels, which can be applied to your face by themselves or mixed with a moisturizer. Try a little bit first and add more if you want more color. Be careful of putting it on your neck if you're wearing light-colored clothing. Make sure to wash your face at the end of the day to prevent buildup in your pores and stains on your pillowcase.

How to Use Sunless Tanning Products

Sunless tanning products can give you a natural-looking tan as long as you know the right way to use them.

Exfoliate First
No matter where you're applying sunless tanner, exfoliate thoroughly first. Removing dead skin cells will ensure a more even result.

Make Sure You're Completely Dry
Applying sunless tanner to dry skin makes it appear more even since water can dilute the product and thereby cause spotting or streaks.

Massage In the Product
Using circular motions, massage the product into the areas you want to tan, making sure to work the product completely into your skin.

Be Careful on Your Joints
Areas like elbows and knees tend to absorb more self-tanner because they are usually drier. Use a light touch on these areas.

Wash Your Hands
After applying the product, wash your hands thoroughly to get all the tanner off. If left on your hands, it can make them look dirty or even orange.

Follow the Directions
Different products take different amounts of time to work. Leave the product on only for the recommended time (which could be anywhere from a few minutes to overnight).

Dry Before Dressing

Make sure to let your body dry completely before getting dressed to decrease the risk of uneven results.

Moisturize Daily

Once the tan has dried, keep your body well hydrated with lotion or cream. The enemy of any tan, natural or sunless, is dehydration.

Get Professional Help

If this sounds too complicated to you, get a professional spray tan instead. Use online review sites and look at before-and-after pictures to find a provider with the best results.

STAY AWAY FROM TANNING BEDS

People used to think indoor tanning was safer than sitting in the sun. Science now tells us that couldn't be more wrong. These beds use highly concentrated UV rays to tan skin more quickly than natural sunlight, and since people who use them rarely use sunscreen, they can damage skin faster than sitting by the pool. In fact, the American Academy of Dermatology says that even one indoor tanning session can exponentially increase your risk of all skin cancers, particularly if you use them before the age of thirty-five. According to the Centers for Disease Control and Prevention, if no one younger than eighteen years old ever used a tanning bed, 61,839 melanomas and 6,735 deaths due to melanoma could be prevented over the lifetime of 61.2 million children. The evidence is so strong that the FDA now requires warning labels on all indoor tanning devices.

WEAR YOUR ART ON YOUR SLEEVE

Tattoos used to be looked down upon as a symbol of rebellion reserved for sailors and motorcycle gangs. Times have changed and tattoos are now not only accepted, but exceedingly common. Reports show that one in four adults in the US has at least one tattoo and that number is steadily rising year over year.

Tattoos at their core are wearable art. They're also personal. A lot of thought is put into getting a tattoo, especially your first, and while the process of getting a tattoo can be painful, getting a tattoo falls into the category of self-care. After all, how often do you put so much thought into altering the appearance of your body? Giving yourself the permission to get a tattoo and actually following through with it takes an amount of care and reflection that stems from self-care motivation. They also require both short- and long-term care in order to keep them looking their best.

First-Timer Tips

Getting your first tattoo is always a daunting experience, but whether you've been thinking about it for years or woke up with a sudden urge to get inked, you should never go into it blind. Follow these steps before going under the needle.

Do Your Research

These days, *Instagram* is the most powerful tool for research when it comes to tattoos. Use it to find styles and artists you like. Most people want their tattoos to have significance, so think about what you want it to look like and find images of similar tattoos to show your artist. Be prepared to articulate to the artist why you want a certain piece and what it means to you.

Find an Artist You Vibe With

Use social media as a tool to find an artist whose work you especially love. Start with hashtags of styles and then go deep in the artist's personal feeds until you get a feel for their style. If social media isn't your thing, ask friends who have tattoos you like for recommendations. Finding the right artist can make all the difference in how happy you are with the results.

Think about Placement

The placement of your tattoo is important, second only to the actual design. If you want to be able to cover it up, think about places on your body you rarely show off. If pain isn't your thing, consider places that are fleshier (since bony areas are more painful to tattoo).

Ask Questions

Most artists will ask for a consultation before tattooing you, especially if you want a custom design. Take this opportunity to ask any questions you have about the process. Come prepared with a deposit (the artist will tell you how much beforehand), and always ask about the final cost.

Keep an Open Mind

Remember that people who tattoo are artists and think of your tattoo as a collaboration. The tattoo artist will always want you to be happy with the result, but they can give you advice on what will look best. They may even have ideas on the design that you haven't even considered. Never try to strong-arm them into doing something they don't want to do; let them be creative, and you'll get a better result.

Be Prepared for Aftercare

Ask about aftercare before you get tattooed. Most reputable tattoo shops will provide you with product samples for aftercare, but it helps to go shopping for ointments and creams beforehand so you're not scrambling after the fact.

Aftercare

Immediate aftercare is a critical time for every tattoo. It can aid the healing process and prevent infection, which can have long-term effects on your health. The first two weeks after getting a tattoo are most critical, but it takes around a month for it to completely heal.

Washing

Wash the tattoo with a gentle, fragrance-free soap to keep the area clean. This should be done a few hours after getting the tattoo and twice a day for about two weeks.

Ointment

Apply a thin layer of healing balm to the tattoo several times a day for the first few days. This will help protect the wounds and facilitate the healing process. The tattooed area will scab over, and once the scabs have completely fallen off, you can switch to lotion.

Lotion

Apply a rich, fragrance-free lotion to the tattoo after the scabs fall off to keep it moisturized and healthy. Hydrated skin is healthy skin and can promote optimal healing as well.

Long-Term Care

No one wants to be that old dude with the saggy tattoo. If you want to keep your tattoo looking fresh for years to come, you have to take special care of it.

Exfoliate

Tattoo ink lives underneath the surface of your skin, which means dead skin buildup can make it look dull. It's especially apparent in tattoos with color, which can fade naturally over time. Removing dead skin cells with exfoliation can help minimize fading. Use a body scrub or chemical exfoliator regularly to keep your skin and tattoos fresh.

Moisturize

Moisturized skin looks healthier and stays tighter, which can help tattoo ink stay vibrant and prevent sagging. Use a daily moisturizer like a body lotion to help keep ink (and skin) looking young. Some people prefer body oils, which they say helps keep the colors in tattoos more vibrant.

Sunscreen

The biggest culprit behind fading tattoos is the sun. It's the same reason the paint on the outside of your house fades over time. The best defense is a good offense by way of wearing daily sunscreen (all over your body is best, but at the very least on your tattoos). It won't entirely prevent fading, but it will slow it down and help guard you against skin cancer at the same time.

Collagen

As you age, your skin naturally loses collagen, which is responsible for keeping it tight and youthful looking. This is why tattoos can warp and change shape over time. It's hard to control this on your body, but one good way to do this is to take ingestible collagen supplements, which, unlike topical applications, distribute the material all over your body.

ABOUT TATTOO REMOVAL

Don't ever get a tattoo with the expectation of removing it later, but regrets can happen. The biggest thing to know before getting a tattoo removed is the darker the ink, the more difficult it is to remove. Tattoos are removed by lasers, which break up dark pigment. Once it's zapped, the pigment is flushed out by your body. It's a slow process and in some cases can take years. Since these lasers target dark pigment, if you have dark skin it can be risky and could leave you with discoloration. Even in the best-case scenario, a tattoo might never be fully removed; you could be left with a scar or a shadow of the ink. If you're serious about tattoo removal, seek out a reputable provider (your dermatologist is a good person to ask for recommendations). In other cases, consider having it covered up with a new one.

GET YOURSELF TO A SPA

For some reason, most guys don't think about spas as realistic tools for their own self-care. Culturally, we see spas as luxury destinations that are meant for occasional pampering. We also see them as almost exclusively feminine: a closed-door refuge where women go to lounge around in towels and get covered in mud (or whatever else they do there). In the minds of many men, spas are scary and weird and uncomfortable.

In reality, spas are totally rad. They're also useful, fun, and yes, relaxing. Everyone should go to a spa at least once in their life, willingly and openly, and it's a guarantee that you'll want to go back.

Spas are like theme parks for self-care. They have it all: facials, massages, steam rooms, even stuff you've never heard of, like floatation chambers and rooms built from Himalayan salt. But like theme parks, they can be the time of your life or completely overwhelming. It depends on what you want to get out of it, and if you do it right, you'll be energized, excited, and aching to go back.

Why Even Go?

To continue with the analogy, your bathroom is like a high school carnival, but a spa is like Disney World. There is no comparison to the level of relaxation you'll get when you're completely immersed in a spa atmosphere. Some people go and they don't even do anything. Most people, however, go to the spa for a specific experience like a massage or a facial. These are things you cannot do yourself. At their core, spas are places where you get services that are the next level up from your own self-care routine.

How to Choose a Spa

The easiest way to choose a spa is to not choose. If you're staying at a hotel with a spa, set aside some time to check it out. These spas are usually straightforward and not very crowded, and if you're a hotel guest, don't cost anything to check out. Go chill in the steam room, or spend some time in the sauna to see if you like the experience.

Most cities and towns have at least one spa somewhere, so look for day spas in your area. Check their websites to see what services and amenities they offer (more on that later) and whether a treatment is required to go. Then check the price list (some spas can be expensive), and look for prices you are comfortable paying within your budget.

Check online reviews to see what other people say about the services. Look especially for comments about the cleanliness of the common areas, the friendliness and professionalism of the staff, and the general atmosphere (how crowded it is, how relaxing the vibe is, etc.). Spa employees should be friendly and make you feel comfortable; when you call to book your appointment, ask them any questions you have, and if it's your first time going to a spa, tell them. They'll be able to give you a tour and answer questions while you're there. And always make sure the therapists and providers are licensed.

What to Do When You're There

The beauty of most spas is that you can get whatever you want out of them. A typical day spa will offer a menu of options from facials to massages to body treatments and sometimes more. Some places will offer amenities like soaking pools, saunas, and steam rooms that you can use even if you're not getting a treatment (this is typical for hotel spas), and some allow you to buy time to use their facilities and just chill. Others require booking a treatment for entry. You'll book a treatment and then be allowed to use the facilities for a set amount of time before or after your treatment.

Most spas are co-ed (though you can find male-only spas if that's more comfortable for you). You'll be shown to a locker room where you'll change into a robe and sandals (check with your spa before you go to see if you need to wear a swimsuit under your robe). Things like single-sex saunas, steam rooms, and showers are located in the locker room. Outside the locker room will usually be a waiting area where you'll await your treatment. Depending on what sort of treatment you're getting, your therapist will bring you back to the appropriate room.

There are also generally communal areas like soaking pools, hot tubs, and other types of saunas and steam rooms. This is usually the area that you are free to use even if you're not getting a treatment. You'll find most people here, lounging around, soaking in the baths, and getting their relaxation on.

Decoding the Spa Menu

Spa treatments can vary widely from location to location, but most spas offer some versions of these basic services. The menu will usually offer an exact description of each service specific to that spa.

Massage

The most iconic spa treatments, massages come in a wide variety like deep tissue, hot stone, Thai, shiatsu, the list goes on. If you've never gotten a massage before, start with a classic Swedish. Most spas will offer you the choice of a male or female therapist.

Facial

It used to be that spas were the only places you could get facials, and they're still the cornerstone of many spa offerings. For more information on why you should get a facial, go to Part 4.

Body Wrap

Body treatments, like wraps, are like facials for your whole body. Most wraps involve the application of moisturizing creams or lotions before you're wrapped up in a sheet or blanket. This helps to facilitate the absorption of the creams deeper into your body, leaving you soft AF.

Body Scrub

Like wraps, scrubs are body treatments. In this case, an exfoliant is applied to your body to remove dead skin cells from head to toe. They're usually followed by a moisturizer.

Manicure/Pedicure

Typically, a manicure or pedicure you'll get at a spa focuses more on moisturizing and relaxation than the one you get at your neighborhood nail salon, but the steps are generally the same.

Amenities

General spa amenities aren't ones you have to book specially. They include steam rooms, saunas, soaking pools, Jacuzzi-style baths, and sometimes even special showers. Consider these extra credit.

NUDE VERSUS NEVER NUDE

One of the things that prevents people from going to spas is the fear of nudity, and truthfully, being naked at some point at the spa is likely. It may just be in the locker room; it may be only during your massage. Other treatments like body scrubs require a bit more nudity. Some spas, especially Korean-style bathhouses, require you be naked in certain areas and baths. In most spas, if you don't want to get naked, you don't have to, but you can't control what other people do, so if nudity makes you uncomfortable, steer clear of those areas. You're there to relax, so don't feel pressure to do something you don't want to do, whether that's wearing clothing or not.

Part 4

FACE

In the Venn diagram of self-care and personal grooming, there is a lot of overlap. Men tend to think of grooming as functional: cleaning yourself so you don't smell, making you hair look presentable enough that you can leave the house, shaving so you don't look like Grizzly Adams (unless you want to look like Grizzly Adams), etc. But grooming is also a way to make yourself feel good. Think about why you choose a certain soap. It's not just about what cleans the best. You also choose soap based on how it smells, how it makes your skin feel after you use it, and maybe even how it looks in your shower.

When you think about self-care, you may think of time-consuming activities like visiting a spa, but the best way to start a self-care practice is to find small, easy things that make you feel good. One of those things could be taking care of your face.

Your face is your calling card. When your face looks good, you have confidence, maybe even swagger. Studies have shown that when people think they look good, it has a real, uplifting effect on their mood and confidence. Anyone who's had a good hair day knows it's true.

HOW TO BUILD A SKINCARE ROUTINE

The majority of men don't take care of their skin the way they should. Some say they don't have time, others don't know what to do, and some say it's girly. These excuses end now. You are allowed to take care of your skin. In fact, you *need* to take care of it. Skin is your body's largest organ and the skin on your face is particularly important since it's exposed to outside elements more often than other parts of your body.

In terms of self-care, a skincare routine is one of the easiest things you can do. It not only helps you look better but also *feel* better. A morning routine can help perk you up as well as a cup of coffee; a nighttime routine can help you wind down.

The most important thing to any skincare routine is to be realistic. Don't overwhelm yourself with too much at once. Start simple. You'll see a difference right away, but the key to any effective skincare routine is consistency.

The Basics

If you are like the majority of guys, you wash your face with water and have never used a moisturizer. If so, here are the first steps you should take to build a skincare routine.

Use a Facial Cleanser

Put down the hand soap. Facial cleansers are designed to clean effectively without disrupting the delicate pH balance of your face. A tight, dry feeling after you wash means the soap was too harsh. A good facial cleanser won't do that. Use your face cleanser morning and night, and more often if you take multiple showers.

What to Get: When in doubt, get something that has the word "gentle" on it. If you know you have a specific skin issue, look for formulas that address it, like a sensitive skin or acne-fighting formula.

Follow with an Eye Cream

The first place most men notice signs of aging is around their eyes (dark circles, bags, and droopy lids). Your best defense is an eye cream. They're super-charged with ingredients to help address all of those things, and even if you're not concerned with wrinkles yet, start using one now. Use an eye cream every time you wash your face.

What to Get: Look for products that contain caffeine, which energizes your skin, and peptides, which are skin-building proteins. If you're not a fan of creams, look for gel formulas.

Finish with a Moisturizer

Dehydrated skin looks dull and sullen, but hydrated skin looks healthier and doesn't age as quickly. Moisturizing is like making sure your gas tank is always full. Use it morning and night after your eye cream.

What to Get: No one likes to feel like their face is covered in goo, so look for a lightweight gel or lotion. If you have oily skin, get an oil-free formula that has the word "matte" on the bottle. Always use a moisturizer that contains SPF if you can find one you like.

A NOTE ON SUNSCREEN

You, as an adult man, know the sun's rays can be harmful to your skin. That's why you (hopefully) wear sunscreen at the beach. The sun is affecting your skin every single day year-round, whether it's sunny or cloudy, and you should wear sunscreen every day. Dermatologists say that they see more aggressive types of skin cancer in men because they don't protect themselves properly. Wearing daily sunscreen is your best defense. The American Academy of Dermatology recommends using minimum SPF 30 and one that is broad spectrum (which means it protects against both UVB and UVA rays). Choose one you can tolerate wearing. After all, the best sunscreen for you is the one you will actually wear.

Advanced Moves

Now that you've mastered a basic skincare routine, there are a few steps you can take to amp up your game.

Level Up with Serum

Serums are like the prize blocks in *Super Mario Bros*. They're tools to help you gain a specific advantage. Serums have concentrated ingredients like vitamin C, which helps to brighten dull skin, or hyaluronic acid, which helps skin retain moisture. Use a serum right after cleansing, morning and night.

What to Get: To start, go for one that targets multiple things. Look for ingredients like hyaluronic acid, vitamin B, and peptides, all of which help improve skin health at a cellular level and are important in skin regeneration.

Exfoliate Smarter

Here's a secret: You're probably exfoliating without knowing it. In the process of shaving, the razor's blade also sloughs away dead skin cells. Exfoliating is important because, as skin cells die, they can accumulate on the surface of your skin and can clog pores. You should exfoliate your whole face regularly, even if you shave, to keep those dead cells in check.

What to Get: Facial scrubs are fine, but they can be harsh on your skin. Instead, use a chemical exfoliant with alpha hydroxy acids (like glycolic acid) to get rid of dead cells more gently.

Night Cream Is the Right Cream

If you want the best skin possible, you should consider using a night cream. During the day, your skin is accosted by aggressors (e.g., sunlight, pollution, dirt), but at night, when your cells aren't busy fighting, they regenerate themselves. Night creams help with this process.

What to Get: Look for a night cream with active ingredients like hyaluronic acid (for hydration), retinol (for anti-aging), or ceramides (for skin tone). If you don't like the feel of heavy cream, try an oil instead.

WHAT I DO: FRANK OCEAN

In an interview with *GQ* in 2019, musician Frank Ocean became the patron saint of night cream. When asked about his skincare routine, he dropped some serious knowledge. "I really do believe in night cream," he said. "You really need to do a gentle wash and put a night moisturizer on. I need the night cream because when I wake up I feel very beautiful, moisturized, and ready to have people making eye contact with me.... That's the life hack right there." So next time you're wondering if a night cream is too extra, remember: If it's good enough for Frank Ocean, it's good enough for you.

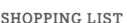

SHOPPING LIST

- **Where to Go:** Great skin care is everywhere; you just have to know where to look. Your local big box or drugstore is a great place to start. Department stores can be intimidating, but they have salespeople who can answer questions. Your best option may be the Internet. Did you know many large online retailers have dedicated men's grooming sections?

- **How Much to Spend:** Some skincare products are expensive, so if you're just starting out, don't shell out a lot. Drugstore products can work just as well as the luxury ones. Facial cleansers, for instance, are easy to save on, while serums and eye creams are worth splurging on.

- **How to Know If Something Is Good:** When shopping online, read user reviews. You'll get a good idea of what other people like. Keep in mind that everyone's skin is different. If you're shopping IRL, ask a salesperson for advice.

- **Make It Easy:** If you don't know where to start, look for boxed sets. Some brands bundle their products into easy-to-use regimens, which allows you to try different products easily.

- **"For Men" Products:** If buying a product that says "For Men" on the label makes you more comfortable, then go for it. But know that what makes most of these products "for men" is the packaging. Don't be afraid to shop the other aisles. Most products are unisex and will work on you too.

- **Try Something New:** Subscription services are easy ways to try new products with little risk. For the same experience in a store, ask for samples before you buy the full-sized product.

SHAVING: THE ORIGINAL MEN'S FACIAL

Shaving is the cornerstone of a man's grooming routine, and maintaining facial hair (or the lack thereof) has been a thing for thousands of years. Around 300 B.C., Alexander the Great required his soldiers to shave their faces clean so enemies couldn't pull their beards in battle. In effect, he set in motion centuries of shaving obsession.

Shaving every day can feel like a chore, and lots of guys think that if they grow a beard, it will be less maintenance than shaving. Spoiler: it's not—but more on that later. The bottom line is that whether you choose to be clean shaven, bearded, or somewhere in between, you're going to spend time dealing with your facial hair. Instead of making it something you begrudge, make it part of your self-care routine. You're already doing it, so here's how to make it an experience you actually look forward to.

The Great Razor Debate

Opinions are strong over what makes the best razor, but the one for you is whatever feels best on your skin. Shaving should not be something that leaves you with a face covered in bandages.

Finding a razor that you can use every day with minimal irritation takes trial and error. To start, you need to know the three main kinds of razors.

Multi-Blade Cartridge Razors

Disposable cartridge razors are easy to use, fairly inexpensive, and widely available. These days, you don't even have to remember to buy them—they show up at your door. Most of these razors have multiple blades, which are thought to give a closer shave. Some people say the more blades on a razor, the more likely you'll get ingrown hairs, since they shave too close.

Single-Blade Safety Razors

In recent years, the old-school single-blade safety razor has come back. Proponents claim they give the best shave for even sensitive skin and help prevent razor bumps and ingrown hairs. They don't cut as close to the skin as a multi-blade razor, which makes it easier for hair to grow back without getting caught. The downside is that "safety" is relative; they're easy to cut yourself with and take some time to get used to.

Electric Razor

The biggest draw of an electric razor is the ease of use. Most are designed to shave your skin while it's dry; they're quick, easy to travel with, and pretty idiot-proof. They may be good for men with sensitive skin because they can be gentler than a classic razor. The downside is they are expensive and you still need to remember to switch out the blades.

How to Shave at Home

Whether your dad taught you how to shave or not, more guys than you'd think say they don't actually know how to shave.

Step 1: Open Up Your Pores
Splash hot water on your face or press a hot towel to your beard area (soak the towel in hot water or zap it in the microwave for a few seconds). Better yet, get in the shower. Hot water and steam will open your pores and soften coarse facial hair.

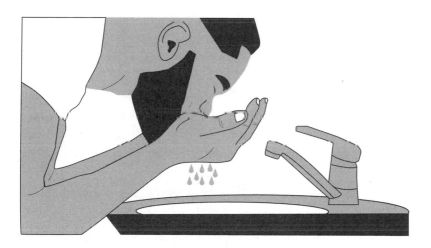

Step 2: Scrub Before You Shave
Dead skin cells can clog the blades of your razor and lead to nicks, so exfoliate before you shave. This also helps hairs stand up so they can be shaved more effectively.

Step 3: Apply a Pre-Shave Oil
Applying an oil before shaving cream helps the razor glide across your skin more easily. If a razor pulls too much, it can lead to razor burn.

Step 4: Use a Moisturizing Shaving Cream

Look for a shaving cream with a rich lather and moisturizing ingredients, which will help cut down on post-shave irritation.

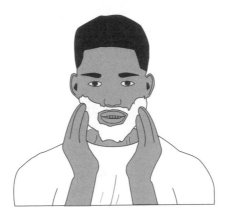

Step 5: Make Sure Your Blade Is Sharp

Dull razors lead to cuts and razor burn because they have to work harder. Make sure your razor is always sharp (most cartridge razors should be changed after about three uses).

Step 6: Shave in the Direction Your Hair Grows

This is called "with the grain." Going against the grain leads to more ingrown hairs and razor bumps.

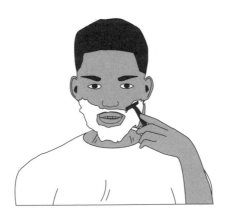

Step 7: Wash Your Face with Cold Water

Rinsing everything off with cold water helps calm your skin after the irritation of shaving and closes pores.

Step 8: Finish with Moisturizer

Apply a post-shave lotion or moisturizer to help seal everything in. It will help calm down your skin and support your skin's natural protective barrier.

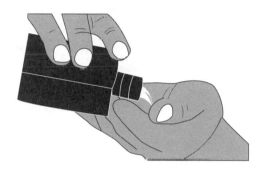

Why Get a Barber Shave?

Before Mr. King Gillette (yes, that's his real name) invented the at-home disposable razor in 1895, the only option men had was to go to the barber. You had to plan in advance and really commit, since a barber shave takes around an hour. But when you're trusting a guy to hold a blade that close to your carotid artery, you don't want to rush him.

These days, there's no reason to get a barber shave, except that it feels damn good. The experience of getting a barber shave is something you can't get at home. Not to mention it's the perfect way to force yourself to unplug even for a few minutes. If you're going to get a barber shave before a special occasion like a wedding, do it the day before in case there is any irritation. Better yet, get one just because—no special occasion needed.

SO YOU DON'T WANT TO SHAVE...

Just because you have a beard doesn't mean you're off the hook for maintenance.

- **Moisturize It:** Hair can become scraggly and the skin underneath can become dry. Massage a moisturizer into the skin underneath and use a beard balm to keep hair hydrated.
- **Wash It:** Beards are way dirtier than you think. Wash your beard with a beard wash often to cleanse the hair and the skin underneath.
- **Trim It:** Invest in an electric trimmer with multiple length settings. To keep the shape of the beard, trim it often so you don't head into ZZ Top territory.
- **Shape It:** See a barber every three to four months. They can freshen up the lines of your beard and trim out the bulk.
- **Shave (Some of) It:** To maintain the lines of your beard, shave your neck and cheeks (and anywhere else there are errant hairs).

SHOPPING LIST

- **Where to Go:** When you're choosing a razor, think about how you're going to get refills. Choose something you can get easily. For shaving creams and aftershave, most men's skincare brands will also have shaving products. A good place to start is a brand you already like.
- **How Much to Spend:** Thanks to online shaving companies, razor refills don't have to set you back a lot. Invest in the best quality razor you can afford and save money on the accoutrements like shaving cream.
- **How to Know If Something Is Good:** If you're looking for a beard trimmer, ask a friend with a spectacular beard or read online reviews. Better yet, ask your barber since he probably does a lot of shaves.
- **Buy for Your Skin Type:** Before buying a new shaving product, know what type of skin you have. If you're prone to breakouts or irritation, use something for sensitive skin or with cooling ingredients like aloe. If you're a man of color, look for brands specifically formulated for your skin, which will help minimize ingrown hairs.
- **Cheaper Isn't Always Better:** Cheap razors get dull faster and sometimes sacrifice shave quality for price. Don't break the bank, but go for something because it makes your skin feel good, not because the price is the lowest.

EVERYTHING YOU NEED TO KNOW ABOUT MASKING

Masking has been an important part of skin care for generations. More recently, thanks to a craze for Korean skincare products, sheet masks have become as ubiquitous as deodorant. You've probably seen your lady friends use them, but if you've never considered using a mask yourself, you're missing out.

Masks are ideal for men who like to use less product and are impatient when it comes to results. These are highly potent and targeted treatments that you use less frequently than other skincare products. They don't replace a regular skincare routine, but if daily skin care is cardio, masking is an interval workout.

Most masks are designed to be used as little as once a week and even with semi-regular use can address skin issues like breakouts, dryness, redness, and oiliness. Most masks fall into five categories and which one you choose depends on the results you want.

Clay Masks

Think of a face mask and you probably conjure an image of a fancy lady with cucumbers on her eyes and a face covered in mud. That's the OG mask—the clay mask. They use ingredients like mud, clay, and charcoal to deep clean pores and cleanse skin in a way that your facial cleanser can't. As the mask dries, it sucks dirt and grime from inside your pores like a vacuum. And can help control shine and breakouts.

How to Use a Clay Mask

Wash your face but don't dry it completely. While your skin is still damp, smear an even layer over your face avoiding your eyes and mouth. Let it dry for around 20 minutes. It may feel tight—that's okay. Wash it off with warm water using your hands or a washcloth. Finish up with a moisturizer.

Peel-Off Masks

Like clay masks, peel-offs are designed to get rid of buildup deep down in your pores. They use sticky ingredients called polymers that attach to grime and pull it out when the mask is removed. They're effective at getting rid of blackheads and controlling shine but can be risky since leaving them on too long can damage your skin barrier. Always follow the directions on the package, and don't leave the mask on for longer than advised.

How to Use a Peel-Off Mask

Wash and dry your face, then apply a thin, even layer of the gel. Avoid your eyes, mouth, eyebrows, and any facial hair. Let the gel dry for the amount of time noted on the bottle (usually around 15–20 minutes), then gently peel it off. Use warm water to clean away any remnants. Follow with a moisturizer to minimize irritation.

Exfoliating Masks

An exfoliating mask will get rid of dead skin cells on the surface of your skin, which can lead to a brighter complexion and help reduce signs of aging. Unlike scrubs, which require you to do the work with your hands, exfoliating masks use acids to break the bonds between dead cells. They require little effort and only need to be used once or twice a week.

How to Use an Exfoliating Mask

Remember that even though they're gentle, these masks still contain acids. Read the directions before using one for the first time and start with a clean face. Some masks stay on for a set amount of time (around 20 minutes) while others are designed to be worn overnight. Whichever one you use, follow with a moisturizer.

Sheet Masks

Sheet masks can be credited with the current masking renaissance, thanks to social media stardom; they look hilarious but also really work. The idea is simple: single-use, disposable masks usually made of paper soaked in serum. As the sheet sits on your face, it creates a barrier that allows the serum to absorb into your skin quickly without evaporating into the air. Sheet masks come in thousands of varieties and most are gentle enough to use every day but once or twice a week is enough.

How to Use a Sheet Mask

After washing your face, tear open the package and unfold the mask. The mask will have holes for your eyes, nose, and mouth. Align these to your face and smooth it down. Keep the mask on your face for around 15–30 minutes, then take if off and throw it away. Gently press any remaining serum into your skin.

Hydrating Masks

When daily moisturizer isn't enough to heal dry skin, like in the depths of winter or after spending the day at the beach, a hydrating mask will bring it back. They're usually a gel or cream and will have ingredients like hyaluronic acid, aloe, and other botanical extracts. Unlike other masks, they can usually be worn for longer periods of time and used more frequently, even every day if you have especially dry or irritated skin.

How to Use a Hydrating Mask

After cleansing, apply a liberal layer to your face, avoiding your eyes. Leave the mask on for the amount of time directed on the bottle. It may not completely dry, but when time is up, wash it off with warm water. Optional: Finish with a moisturizer for extra hydration.

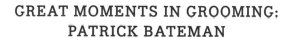

GREAT MOMENTS IN GROOMING: PATRICK BATEMAN

One of the most iconic moments in male grooming is the morning routine of Patrick Bateman in *American Psycho*. Meant to represent the epitome of eighties narcissism, by today's standards it seems pretty tame. His "extensive" routine features an ice pack to depuff his eyes while he does crunches, a deep-pore-cleansing lotion and exfoliating gel scrub in the shower, followed by an herbal mint facial mask that he leaves on for 10 minutes. The rest is an alcohol-free aftershave, two moisturizers, and eye cream. Compared to skincare routines in 2019, it's really pretty standard, except for maybe the peel-off mask. Using a peel-off mint mask every day could actually have a drying effect on his skin, even with his dual moisturizer situation. Maybe a sheet mask instead with an exfoliating mask thrown in there once a week? Just a suggestion.

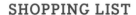

SHOPPING LIST

- **Where to Go:** We're living in the golden age of masking, and they're available almost everywhere: from your grocery store to your local big box. They're also readily available online.
- **How Much to Spend:** The good thing about masks, especially sheet masks, is that they're pretty cheap. The risk factor is low, so try an inexpensive one. If masking becomes part of your normal routine, consider investing a bit more.
- **How to Know If Something Is Good:** We can thank social media for masking's popularity, so that's a good place to start. Look at what mask you see people using on apps and websites like *Instagram*, and try it for yourself. When buying on the Internet, always read reviews.
- **Look for Multipacks:** The low price tag of many sheet masks means they don't cost much, but you only get one use. Look for multipacks, which cost more up front but are discounted in the long run.

FACIALS: CHECKING UNDER THE HOOD

As self-care practices go, facials check all the boxes. They're relaxing and require you to power down and leave your phone alone. They're also practical and help increase the efficacy of your daily skincare routine. Think of it this way: Your car might run fine if you don't take it to a mechanic, but it could run a lot better if you did. Facials are like letting a professional check under the hood.

Facials tend to get overlooked in male grooming. A lot of guys think of them as fussy and luxurious, and many don't want to take the time out of their schedules to get one. That's not an excuse anymore. These days, facials are as easy to get as a haircut. In fact, that's exactly how you should think of them. Experts say that you should get a facial at least four times a year at the change of the seasons. Seasonal changes can affect your skin in different ways (like a whole summer's worth of sweat-clogged pores) and getting a facial is a way to push the reset button on your face.

Facials are also valuable learning experiences. They won't replace your daily skincare routine, but a professional will be able to assess how well it's working and offer you advice on what to do better. They're the mechanics in this ongoing analogy.

In terms of self-care, don't discount the self-esteem bump you get from walking out of a facial with a fresh face. Your face will be brighter and clearer and you won't be able to resist checking it out in every shiny surface you pass. So what are you waiting for?

What to Expect from a Facial

To the uninitiated, facials can seem like a lot of effort just for something you can do at home. But you can't do this at home. A professional can see things you can't, has solutions to problems that you didn't even know existed, and can anticipate future issues (and prevent them). Before you sit down for your first facial, here's how they work.

Step 1: Cleansing
Your aesthetician will start by cleansing your face, often twice, to make sure they have a clean slate to work with.

Step 2: Inspection
Next, they'll look at your skin under a bright light, assessing the situation and formulating a game plan.

Step 3: Exfoliation
Depending on your needs, they'll usually use some sort of exfoliation. This could mean an enzyme peel, a facial scrub, or something stronger depending on how sensitive your skin is and how much exfoliation you need.

Step 4: Extractions
Even if breakouts aren't an issue for you, your aesthetician may advise on extractions. This is when they manually (with their fingers or a tool) extract debris and dirt from your pores. An aesthetician is trained in how to pop zits, push out blackheads, and clear

your skin safely so it won't leave long-term marks. Extractions can sometimes hurt, so your aesthetician will sometimes give you the option to opt out.

Step 5: Mask

Following extractions, your skin usually needs to be calmed down. Your aesthetician will usually use a soothing, hydrating serum and a mask to re-moisturize your skin and minimize irritation.

Step 6: Treatments

After the mask will come more serums and treatments depending on what your skin's needs are. There could be additional tools besides products, like oxygen or LED lights.

Step 7: Moisturizer/SPF

At the end, the aesthetician will prepare your skin for going back out in the world. This usually means locking everything in with a moisturizer and applying an SPF if you're getting the facial during daylight hours.

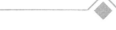

DECODING THE SERVICE MENU

Most facials follow the same general steps, but depending on where you go, there may be additional services offered. The best thing to do is sit back and trust your facialist; they know what your skin needs in order to look its best. When you're booking your first facial, go for something basic and then ask about add-ons later.

These are some common treatments you may encounter.

- **Oxygen:** Pure oxygen can kill bacteria deep in your pores and balance skin on the surface. It also helps to soothe irritated skin.
- **Microcurrent:** These devices use electricity to stimulate facial muscles below the surface. It's a way to tighten and tone your face, so this technology is often found in anti-aging facials.
- **Radiofrequency:** Similar to microcurrent, radiofrequency uses radio waves to stimulate collagen production and tighten skin. It is said to offer an immediate lifting effect and also aid in collagen production for weeks after the treatment.
- **Lymphatic massage:** Your lymphatic system is like your body's plumbing; it helps to flush out waste and keep everything moving. Facial, or lymphatic, massage is a way to stimulate flow, decrease puffiness, and get rid of bloating.
- **LED light therapy:** Studies have shown that certain colors of LED lights have effects on your skin with continued use. Red helps decrease irritation, and blue has an antibacterial effect and can help control acne. Finishing a facial with a few minutes of LED therapy is common.
- **Microdermabrasion:** Think of this as a super scrub. Tiny particles, much smaller than the beads in your at-home facial scrub, exfoliate dead skin cells gently and effectively. This treatment also has been shown to help minimize the look of fine lines and wrinkles over time.

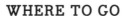

WHERE TO GO

For most men, the biggest obstacle to getting a facial is actually setting foot in the spa. Traditionally, facials were a luxury service that you could only get in a fancy spa, and most men don't want to take the time to sit around in a robe. These days, however, there are things called facial bars. They're no-frills places that typically only offer facials and are quick and easy (you don't even have to change clothes). They're ideal for maintenance and many even offer monthly memberships so a facial can become part of your regular grooming routine.

The most important thing in getting a facial is making sure you're comfortable. Take into account the price—don't cheap out, but don't feel you have to break the bank either. Find a place that's convenient and where you like the vibe—you should feel excited to go. Find an aesthetician you want to see on a regular basis—the more an aesthetician sees your skin, the better they can assess what is going on and anticipate problems before they arise. And by no means are you locked in to one place if you don't like it—try a few different places in order to find the best for you.

FIX YOUR TEETH, FIX YOUR LIFE

It's simple: When you're happy, you smile more, putting your pearly whites (or not so pearly whites) on display. Studies have shown that how your teeth look can actually impact your self-esteem and mood. It's actually been found that people who suffer from depression neglect their oral hygiene. Conversely, those who are happy with how their teeth look smile more and are perceived as happier and friendlier.

Oral hygiene as a self-care practice can have wide-reaching effects. However, when talking about taking care of your face, the importance of your teeth tends to get overlooked. Let's stop that now. Good dental hygiene will not only keep you healthier in the long run but also happier (and can even keep you looking younger).

Tenets of Good Dental Hygiene

Anyone who has been to the dentist before knows what they should do to take care of their teeth. Whether they actually do it is a different story. Some studies show that only around 64 percent of American adults visit the dentist once a year and 23 percent have gone two or more days without brushing their teeth. Building a consistent oral hygiene practice is the first step to long-term health and creating a better-looking smile. This is how to do it.

Brush Twice a Day
The American Dental Association (ADA) says everyone should brush their teeth in the morning and before bed for 2 full minutes (the average person falls short in both frequency and time).

Use a Toothpaste with Fluoride
No matter what kind of toothpaste you use, make sure it contains fluoride, an ingredient shown to help strengthen teeth and prevent cavities. Even a natural toothpaste should contain fluoride for optimal dental health.

Floss after You Brush
Flossing every time after you brush your teeth is known to reduce decay, prevent cavities, and help fight gum disease. Some surveys show that only 40 percent of adults floss their teeth every day. Don't be part of the other 60 percent. If you have a hard time flossing or your gums are sensitive, consider using a water flosser.

Use an Alcohol-Free Mouth Rinse
Not all dentists endorse mouthwashes, but using one once a day can help kill bacteria that live in the mouth and help prevent bad breath. Look for formulas that don't contain alcohol, which can be drying.

Try Tongue Scraping
Ayurvedic medicine believes in the benefits of daily tongue scraping. It's not as popular in Western cultures, but if you really want to level up your dental hygiene, consider adopting the habit.

Your Toothbrush Matters

Your oral hygiene is only as good as the tools you use; the right toothbrush is the most important in your kit. According to the

ADA, both manual and electric toothbrushes can be effective, provided you use them to brush for 2 minutes twice a day. However, many dentists know the likelihood of the average person doing that is pretty low. For that reason, they sometimes recommend electric toothbrushes to get rid of plaque and bacteria with minimal effort and user error.

The benefit of an electric toothbrush is that it takes out guesswork. Most have automatic timers that automatically shut off after 2 minutes. They are also able to break up plaque in hard-to-reach places, like between teeth, quicker than manual toothbrushes can. Some models even automatically remind you to switch the brush head when it's time to change it (which, for the record, is every three to four months). The downside is that these toothbrushes can be expensive. If you can afford it, consider upgrading, but if you can't, don't sweat it. The best toothbrush for you is the one you'll actually use.

At-Home Whitening

Most people just want their smile to be whiter. White teeth are a sign of good health, look more youthful, and make a smile look wider and brighter. Taking care of your teeth on a daily basis can help teeth be whiter (by removing surface stains), but most people want a little extra. That's why at-home whitening products are so popular. These are some of the most common ways to whiten your smile.

Whitening Toothpaste
Whitening toothpaste contains tiny abrasive ingredients that physically scrape away stains as you brush. Dentists recommend against using whitening toothpaste every day, since those same abrasive ingredients can weaken enamel with overuse. As an

alternative, consider whitening toothpastes that contain hydrogen peroxide or apple cider vinegar, which can help remove stains.

Stick-On Strips

These strips are coated in a bleaching agent and then stick to your teeth for a set amount of time. Consistent use has shown they lighten the color of teeth effectively and safely. Dentists like these because they're mild and aren't as harsh on your teeth (with correct use).

LED Light Therapy

LED light therapy has recently become popular for teeth whitening when used in combination with bleaching gels. The light helps the bleach work better and penetrate deeper. It also is thought to be better for sensitive teeth and gums.

Whitening Pen

These products are like spot treatments for your teeth. They're like markers: The paintbrush-like tip is soaked in a bleaching agent, and you apply it directly to your teeth to address specific stains. They're ideal for travel or if you want to address a specific tooth.

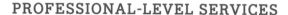

PROFESSIONAL-LEVEL SERVICES

There's plenty you can do to improve your smile at home, but if you want to change the game, it's best to see your dentist. Most dentists offer professional-level cosmetic treatments that provide results you can't get with over-the-counter products.

- **Professional whitening:** Think of this as the monster truck of light-based whitening treatments. This quick treatment uses a combination of peroxide and LED light to lighten your teeth several shades in just one go. The downside is that some patients have reported increased sensitivity and pain directly after the treatment. Plus, it can run you several hundred dollars per session. The upside? One treatment can last you a year.
- **Orthodontics:** Besides the color, one of the biggest issues people have with their teeth is how straight they are. Even if you had braces when you were a kid, teeth keep moving your whole life due to gradual soft tissue and bone loss. To get your teeth back in line, consider invisible aligners, which help straighten your teeth through a series of invisible trays. They're more adult-friendly than braces.
- **Veneers:** If traditional orthodontics are a road trip, veneers are traveling in a private jet. Veneers are thin, false teeth that fit over your existing ones. It used to be that to get veneers, you had to permanently damage your natural teeth, but new technology allows veneers to be placed without completely getting rid of the teeth underneath. They typically cost several thousand dollars per tooth, and need to be replaced every fifteen to twenty years, but nothing else comes close to really changing your smile.

ANTI-AGING: START BEFORE IT'S TOO LATE

It's often said that, like fine wines, men look better with age; we use words like *rugged* and *distinguished* to describe dudes who look a little more mature. Double standards aside, there's a fine line between looking mature and looking old. No one wants to look old.

The fact that many men don't have much of an anti-aging routine seems fine until it's not. Men tend to neglect themselves, and they start addressing aging when it's too late. The most important thing to know about anti-aging is you have to start early. There is no magic product that will completely erase wrinkles once they've formed, but a good skincare routine with the right ingredients will help slow their appearance so you don't wake up one morning looking like a raisin.

For better or worse, women are taught to start taking steps to prevent the appearance of aging from an early age and spend most of their lives trying to prevent it. Men need to take a page from that book and train themselves to be proactive instead of reactive. Men worry about aging just as much as women do; they just don't talk about it. And by not talking about it, they aren't as prepared.

As people age, their skin gradually decreases its production of collagen, the substance that keeps skin tight and firm. They also lose fat in their faces, which, coupled with looser skin, means that wrinkles form and skin sags. In men, this most often starts to show around the eyes and around the chin and neck. Lines may become etched in the forehead and between the brows, which comes from years of furrowing. Skin may become drier and redness can become an issue.

None of this should scare you necessarily. Aging isn't a bad thing; it's a fact of life. Self-care is about giving yourself what you need; taking care of yourself has thousands of benefits, and reducing signs of age could be one, if that's what you're hoping for. An anti-aging-focused skincare routine isn't just about trying to stop aging. Proper steps will make your skin look better in general, wrinkles or not. The first is creating a sustainable daily skincare routine. The next step is incorporating some of the following.

Exfoliation

By now you know what exfoliation is and why it's important, but it becomes even more important as you get older. The aging process slows down the rate at which your skin cells regenerate. On average, it takes about twenty-eight days for cells to turn over; as you get older, this timeline gets longer. As a result, dead skin cells stick around on the surface of your skin, which can lead to dryness, rough patches, and uneven skin tone. Your skin can also become more sensitive, which means that the facial scrub you've been using may turn out to be too harsh. Instead, use a chemical exfoliant regularly. Look for products containing alpha hydroxy acids like glycolic or lactic acid, as well as beta hydroxy acids like salicylic acid. Both types of acids help to gently dissolve the bonds that attach dead skin cells to your face and move them along without scrubbing. Some products are gentle enough to use every day, but if you've never used one before, start with once or twice a week and work your way up.

Moisturize

Moisturizing is the cornerstone to any skincare routine, and it only gets more important as you get older. The aging process means that as skin loses its ability to produce collagen, it also decreases its ability to retain moisture. Dry skin is duller, thinner looking, and more easily etched with fine lines and wrinkles. Using moisturizer daily can help with this, and as you get older, you may need to use heavier creams that help hydrate deeply and lock in moisture. Look for products that contain hyaluronic acid, a naturally occurring substance that helps cells retain water, and ceramides, which help form a protective layer to prevent loss of moisture.

Vitamin C

Signs of aging in the skin have been linked to things called free radicals, which can be caused from sun exposure, environmental pollution, and even your diet, and damage healthy cells (scientifically speaking, they steal electrons from other molecules). The best way to combat free radicals is with antioxidants, of which vitamin C is king. Just like you use vitamin C to strengthen your immune system inside your body, it can help strengthen skin when used in your skincare products. Vitamin C prevents oxidative stress caused by free radicals and can brighten skin, promote a more even skin tone, help lighten sun spots and hyperpigmentation, and even prevent lines and wrinkles from getting deeper. The best way to use it is to integrate a serum into your routine (apply it to your face after cleansing and before using moisturizer).

Retinol

According to dermatologists, retinol is one of the most important ingredients you should be using in your skin care, whether you're concerned with aging or not. That's because this form of vitamin A has been studied for decades and has been shown to help with everything from aging to acne and may even prevent some forms of skin cancer. The secret is how it works: Retinol works below the surface of your skin to promote cell turnover and keep the regenerative timeline on track. Remember how the life cycle of your skin cells slows down as you age? Retinol helps prevent that. If you've struggled with acne you may already be using it (it's the active ingredient in many prescription acne products). If you're not, start now. Retinol can be irritating to your skin, especially when first using it, so start slow and apply it after cleansing at night once a week. Work up to using it every night. Retinol can also make your skin more sensitive to sun, so only apply it at night and wear sunscreen during the day.

Sunscreen

Most dermatologists agree that sunscreen not only helps prevent skin cancer, but it's also one of the most effective anti-aging remedies available. This is because damage from UV rays has been linked to nearly every form of aging from wrinkles to sagging skin. It's because of those free radicals mentioned earlier; they are caused by sun exposure and have the ability to wreak havoc on your skin at a cellular level. Sunscreen is your best defense and should be worn daily. If you haven't already, start now.

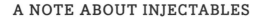

A NOTE ABOUT INJECTABLES

Statistics show that for the last decade, men have made an ever-increasing percent of injectable patients (Brotox, anyone?). But even though the number of men doing it is growing, they're not talking about it. The fact is that getting Botox or a filler is much more common than you assume. There is no shame in going under the needle. Botox and other neuromodulators work by freezing the muscles below the skin so they don't move as much and create wrinkles. Dermal fillers, on the other hand, fill in volume where it is lost through the aging process. Before you make the leap, do your research; a good place to start is your dermatologist. Read online review sites, and look at before-and-after pictures from local practitioners. Always get a consultation before getting injected for the first time, and never make the decision on where to go by price alone.

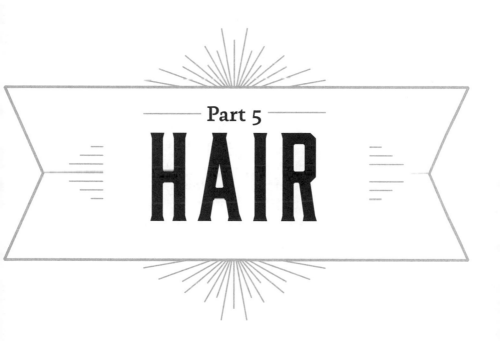

Part 5

HAIR

No matter what kind of hair you have (or how much of it you have), everyone wants great hair. It's part of the human experience, and like it or not, your hair says a lot about you. Humans have always attached importance to hair (hello, Samson) and have always spent an exorbitant amount of time styling, cutting, coloring, and caring for it.

Studies have shown that how you feel about your hair has a real effect on your mood. The Good Hair Day Effect means that when you think your hair looks good, like right after leaving the barber or when you do an especially good job styling it, your posture actually changes, you smile more, you are friendlier to other people, and you have more confidence. Everyone has experienced this at some point—it's that feeling when you catch your reflection in a mirror and think, "Damn, I look good."

That exact phenomenon is why hair care falls under the umbrella of self-care. It's not just about treating your hair well so it's healthy or making your hair look good on the outside. It's also about how your hair makes you feel on the inside and how it can impact your life in a positive way. After all, as self-care teaches you, if it doesn't make you feel good, why do it?

THROW OUT THE 3-IN-1

Every great head of hair starts with how it's taken care of. Men think of hair care as part of an in shower checklist to get through as quickly as possible. That's why multiuse products are so popular: Product developers and marketers believed for a long time that the only way to get men to use hair products was to consolidate them into one.

Spoiler alert: Products that you wash your body with are not the right ones for your hair. Using the right products can not only make your hair look better and be easier to style, but it may also help you keep more of it down the road. Think of taking care of your hair as not just improving what's on your head but your life in general. And it all starts with what you do in the shower.

How to Take Care of Your Hair

You may think hair care boils down to making sure it's clean, but it's more than that. Proper hair care means that your hair not only looks better, but that it's healthier too. Plus, it could also help you keep more of it.

Don't Use Multiuse Products

Multiuse products, like shampoo/conditioner combos and hair/body/face washes, are still popular and sound great...on paper. But conditioning your hair is an important part of hair care (more on that later). The problem with these products is that they do a lot of things okay but nothing particularly well. In the case of shampoo/conditioner combos, they shampoo better than they condition so leave your hair stripped and dry. Instead, use separate shampoos and conditioners or, if your hair is curly, a cleansing conditioner.

Don't Shampoo Every Day

Even if your hair is very short, washing your hair every day can make your hair dry and brittle. Traditional shampoos clean your hair and scalp with soap that strips away the natural oils from your scalp. These oils serve to nourish, moisturize, and protect your hair naturally. The most you should be washing your hair is every other day, and many men can go even longer (like once a week). If you are very active or sweaty or your hair gets greasy fast, use a shampoo that's sulfate-free. It won't strip away as much oil with each use.

Use the Right Shampoo

To the cynic, special shampoos based on your hair type might sound like marketing mumbo jumbo, but they actually exist for a reason. Different hair types have different needs and these special shampoos have ingredients to address them. Thin hair can get pumped up with volumizing shampoo, for instance, thanks to hair-building proteins, and shampoos for curly hair, which tends to get dry quickly, have more moisturizing ingredients.

Always Use Conditioner

Since shampooing strips natural oils from your hair, conditioning is an important step in replenishing that lost moisture. Even if you have short hair, you should use a conditioner every time you shampoo. It's especially important for medium to long hair, since the longer your hair is, the more easily it dries out (oil has a harder time reaching the tips). Even on days when you don't shampoo, you should condition your hair. A good rule of thumb is the more hair you have, the more conditioner you need.

Massage When You Shampoo

No truly great head of hair can exist without a healthy scalp. Just like your face, the skin on your scalp needs to be cared for, and part of this care is exfoliation. Every time you shampoo, use your fingertips and nails to gently massage your scalp. This will not only help the shampoo clean your scalp but will also stimulate blood flow and gently slough away dead skin.

Use a Scalp Scrub

Think of it this way: Your scalp is a garden and your hair is the plants. If the soil is covered in debris, the plants have a harder time poking through. Use a scalp scrub about once a week to make sure all the debris is cleared and the soil is primed for optimal growth. Most scrubs double as shampoos, but if you use one that doesn't, use it before you shampoo.

Dry Hair Gently

Hair should be treated gently, no matter how much you have (if your hair is thinning, it deserves an extra-fine touch). Wet hair is delicate and can break more easily, so after your shower, use the towel to gently pat your hair dry instead of rubbing. It will help keep the strands intact and preserve the natural texture too.

Decoding the Bottle

Out of all the personal grooming products out there, shampoo bottles can have the most confusing jargon. This is what those terms actually mean.

Sulfate-Free
Sulfates are chemicals found in cleansing products that make them lather. People have been trained to expect lather from soap, but many believe sulfates are responsible for overly stripping oil from hair. Most experts these days recommend sulfate-free shampoo.

Paraben-Free
All grooming products contain preservatives that allow them to sit on store and bathroom shelves for long periods of time without going bad. Parabens have been used as preservatives for generations but have come under fire because some believe they are linked to cancer (the medical evidence to support this has not been found).

Phthalate-Free
These chemicals are responsible for creating gel textures in grooming products as well as making artificial fragrances last longer. They're considered endocrine disruptors, which means they may be linked to certain forms of cancer.

Silicone-Free
Silicone is used in grooming products to create "slip," that smooth feeling you get after using some conditioners and lotions. Proponents say it creates a protective coating on hair that allows it to stay smoother longer and keep damage at bay. Critics say it can suffocate hair and actually do more harm than good.

Anti-Dandruff
Dandruff is caused by a fungus that grows on your scalp, and true anti-dandruff shampoos contain antifungal ingredients like zinc pyrithione and ketoconazole. They're great at controlling actual dandruff but won't do much if your itchiness and flakes are caused by something else. Before switching to dandruff shampoo, speak to your dermatologist.

SHOPPING LIST

- **Where to Go:** You can get quality shampoos and conditioners wherever you're already shopping: the supermarket, the drugstore, the big-box store, or online. It doesn't matter where you're buying it as long as it's not a multiuse product and it's specific for your hair type.
- **How Much to Spend:** Buying on a budget is totally cool; when you're using something as often as shampoo, you don't need to feel pressure to shell out more than you can afford. Take the price tag into account, but also make sure it's sulfate-free and has quality ingredients that won't damage your hair.
- **How to Know If Something's Good:** You won't know if you like something until you've actually tried it. If it makes your hair feel too squeaky clean, it's not good. Buy a travel size first, so you're not committing to the family-sized bottle right off the bat. And if you're buying online, reviews are invaluable, but take them with a grain of salt—everyone's hair is different.
- **Ask an Expert:** Your barber works with hair all day and is your best resource for product recommendations. They'll be able to advise on a good shampoo and conditioner for your specific hair type. If you are worried about dandruff or thinning, ask your dermatologist what they would recommend to help control it.
- **"For Men" Products:** If a product that says it's "For Men" makes you feel better keeping it in the shower, that's fine. Just make sure it isn't a multiuse product and that it doesn't contain any harsh ingredients like charcoal. Remember, hair should be treated gently.

YOU SHOULD BE USING A HAIR DRYER

There's a scene in the movie *Saturday Night Fever* where Tony Manero, played by John Travolta, is getting ready to go out. His routine centers on his hair, particularly getting it big and poofy with a blow dryer. Decades later, it remains one of the most recognizable men's grooming moments in pop culture. Whether or not you're old enough to remember it isn't the point. It's that Tony understood how important a blow dryer was in achieving the look he wanted ("Watch the hair!").

That's something your barber or hairstylist also knows and is why they use a blow dryer at the end of your haircut. See, hair dryers are used for more than just cleaning hair off your neck; they shape your hair, help products work better, and yes, help it dry faster. A blow dryer is one of the most important tools in a professional hairstylist's arsenal, and it should be in yours too. A blow dryer can change the game for even short hair, and, let's get real, if there is a tool that will get you out the door faster in the morning, why aren't you using it?

If you don't own a hair dryer, try using one at the gym to get a feel for it. Then buy an inexpensive one and try it out at home. Dryers can cost into the triple digits, but unless you're a professional stylist or are going for an intricate quaff, a basic version will work just fine. As for how to use it? Here's what you need to know.

Parts of a Hair Dryer

Most hair dryers are made up of the same basic components, even the cheapest ones. The more you pay, the more bells and whistles you'll get, and whether you need to use them is up to you.

Heat Setting

Hair dryers commonly have three heat settings: low, medium, and high. These allow you to control how much heat is being blown onto your hair and scalp.

Fan Setting

Like the heat settings, many hair dryers come with multiple fan settings, which allow you to control how fast the air is moving. If yours doesn't, it's not as important as the heat settings. If yours does, keep it on medium or low (the high setting may cause frizz more easily).

Concentrator

When you buy a hair dryer, it may come with a few attachments. A common one is the concentrator, which is like an end cap with a slit in it. This forces the air through a smaller area, allowing you to control where it's going more easily and target specific areas of the hair. It's particularly useful for styles like pompadours, which depend on a lot of volume in the front.

Diffuser

Less common than concentrators, a diffuser is an attachment meant to mimic air drying by dispersing air into a larger area (like the opposite of a concentrator). These are used for curly hair, to preserve the natural texture of hair without frizzing it out, but still drying it quickly.

Cold Button

Most dryers will have a cold button, which turns off the heater and allows cold air to lock in the style once hair is dry.

Using a Hair Dryer

If you've never used a hair dryer, it can be intimidating, especially if your only interaction with them is at the barber when they do a bunch of fancy-looking stuff. In practice, it's pretty simple. Just follow these steps.

Step 1: Comb Out Tangles

While your hair is still damp, run a comb or brush through to get rid of any tangles. While you're doing that, start moving it into the general shape you want.

Step 2: Apply Product to Wet Hair

Some products like gels, salt sprays, and water-based pomades are meant to be applied on damp hair. Use a dime-sized amount and work it through all of your hair. Shape it into the style you want. As you blow dry, the product will activate.

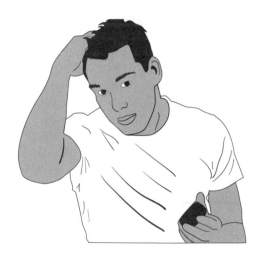

Step 3: Don't Hold It Too Close to Your Head

Hair dryers can get as hot as 140ºF, which means they actually can burn your scalp (and damage hair in the process). Always hold the dryer about 6 to 8 inches away from your head.

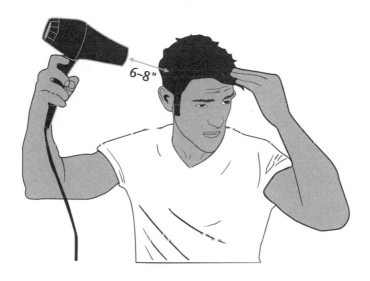

6–8"

Step 4: Use It to Direct the Hair

The point of a hair dryer isn't just to dry your hair but to shape it as it dries. Point the nozzle of the dryer in the direction you want your hair to go and let the air push it, like to get your bangs up and away from your face. If your hair dries in a certain shape, it will stay that way longer.

Step 5: Use a Brush

As you direct the air, you might want to use a brush to keep your hair in place. Holding your hair in position with a barber brush or round brush will help lock in the shape and make sure the roots dry quickly, which helps with volume.

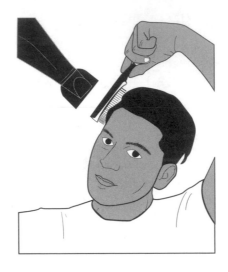

Step 6: Don't Overuse It

The downside to a hair dryer is that there is such a thing as heat damage; too much heat can make hair dry and brittle. Once your hair is dried how you want it, turn the dryer off. Drying it too much is counterproductive.

HOW TO HACK THE HAIR DRYER

While using a hair dryer is simple, these are some pro-level tips that can make the experience (and results) even better.

- **Use the Cold Setting:** Remember that cold setting we talked about before? It actually serves a function. When hair is dried with heat, it becomes malleable but stays that way for a bit even after the dryer is turned off. Once your hair is dry, use the cold setting to blast it with cool air. It will lock everything in place and help your style last.

- **High Heat Is Not Always the Best Heat:** Men tend to think that more is better, but that's not always the case. High heat is okay for healthy hair, but most guys can stick with the medium setting. If you have fine or thin hair, use the low setting to help preserve and volumize it.
- **Flip Your Head to Dry Underneath:** If you have longer hair, flip your head upside down and use the blow dryer to get the hairs underneath. It will not only get them dry but help pump up the volume of this area, which can tend to get flat.
- **Use Your Fingers to Get Texture:** If you're going for a messy, textured look, use your fingers to shape your hair instead of a brush. Brushes will help smooth and shape hair, sure, but give a more polished look. Use your fingers the same way to control the direction and shape, but with a messier result.

HAIR PRODUCTS AND HOW TO USE THEM

Hair care is the first step to a truly great head of hair, but it doesn't stop there. Styling is the other piece of the puzzle. Styling products are helpful, but they're also endlessly confusing, thanks to the sheer variety of them. Knowing what products do is one thing; knowing how to use them is another.

Ask any professional hairstylist and they will tell you that almost every man who actually uses products uses too much. The other mistake men make is using product to force hair into submission. Styling products are meant to enhance the hair you have without completely altering its appearance.

Let's get real: How your hair looks is what you truly care about. That's why styling your hair is as important an act of self-care as making sure it's healthy. Products are tools to make your hair look its best, like wearing a well-fitting suit. Here's how to get the most out of them.

Types of Hair Products

Choosing the right hair product depends on the result you want and the hair type you have.

Pomade

Pomade used to be oil-based, but now is usually water-based and comes in untold varieties. It's the most versatile and well-suited product for most men's hair.

What it does: It's best for parting the hair and slicking. Matte versions are best for messier looks.

Clay

It's like pomade but has no shine, and it leaves a dry, natural finish.

What it does: The dryness creates separation in the hair and increases texture and is best for messy looks.

Wax

Usually it's literal wax and is heavy, shiny, and, well, waxy.

What it does: It has more shine than pomade and offers a lot of control. It's also ideal for creating shape in coarse and textured hair since it locks in moisture without sacrificing hold.

Paste

Paste is creamier than pomade and has less hold but is also more moisturizing, which makes it ideal for curly or wavy hair.

What it does: It leaves a natural finish that's not shiny. It's good for adding texture to styles that are a bit longer.

Gel

Traditionally, gel is used when you want a lot of shine and for your hair to never move. It's contributed to generations of bad hair (Gordon Gekko, anyone?), but modern gels are lighter weight.

What it does: As it dries, it creates a coating on the hair and keeps it in the shape you style it in. It's also used to define curls and protect them from frizz.

Cream

Cream looks like lotion and helps keep hair hydrated and healthy. It's especially ideal for curly or wavy textured hair, but works on anyone.

What it does: Smooths hair and keeps its natural texture but still holds it in place. It's best for natural looks, like you're not wearing product at all.

Salt Spray

Barbers used to mix table salt and water to achieve a fresh-off-the-beach look. Modern salt sprays have healthy oils and natural salt, which add texture without over-drying.

What it does: The salt creates texture that lends a piecey surfer look without the weight of a paste or pomade. It's also ideal for thinning hair since it's non-greasy but adds lots of volume.

Hair Spray

It locks in your style and protects it throughout the day. New versions offer lots of hold but with not as much crunch as the old ones.

What it does: It forms a protective barrier against heat, wind, your open car window, everything. Start with a light dusting to prevent helmet head.

How to Use Products

Ask any hairstylist and they'll tell you that most men don't use hair product correctly. Here's how to not be one of those guys.

Step 1: Start with Damp Hair

Most products these days are water soluble, which means they'll be easier to apply if your hair is damp. Unless the package says specifically to apply on dry hair, apply it onto towel-dried hair and then use a hair dryer.

Step 2: Use the Right Amount

No matter what product you're using, start with a pea- to dime-sized amount. You can always add more product into your hair if you need it, but the only thing to do if you put in too much is to get back in the shower.

Step 3: Cover Your Hands

Rub your hands together to make sure your entire palms are covered. Work the product between your fingers, which you'll be using to shape your hair.

Step 4: Start in the Back

Start rubbing the product into your hair at the back and work your way forward. Starting at the back ensures a more even application (and you can always add more in the front if you need it).

Step 5: Cover, Then Shape

As you're applying, make sure to really distribute the product through all of your hair. Once it's massaged in, go back and shape it into the style you want.

Step 6: Use Hair Spray Last

Once your style is completely dry, lock it in with hair spray. You can either spray it directly on your hair (lightly) or spray it onto a brush and run it through your hair.

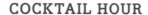

COCKTAIL HOUR

Most professional barbers and hairstylists know something you don't: To really get a good look, you need to use more than one product. To really achieve the look you want, you may need to open yourself up to some cocktails. These are some tried-and-true combos to help your hair look even better.

- **Styling Cream + Matte Pomade = Messy Bedhead:** Use a styling cream for a little hold then apply matte pomade to add texture and cut down on any shine from the cream.
- **Volumizing Spray + Pomade = Thin Hair Antidote:** While your hair is still wet, spray on a volumizing spray to pump up the strands, then apply a small amount of pomade to create the shape.
- **Lightweight Gel + Hair Spray = A Better Part:** Apply a lightweight gel to damp hair, then use a hair dryer and brush to create the shape, then lock it in with hair spray.

SHOPPING LIST

- **Where to Go:** Start with the place where you buy your shampoo or other grooming products. If you have a brand of shampoo you already like, look to see if they also make styling products. If you're shopping online, pay attention to the similar products recommended based on what you're buying.
- **How Much to Spend:** Paying more for a product doesn't necessarily mean it's going to work better. Don't get too hung up on prices. If you want to try something new, get an inexpensive version to see if you like the experience and results.
- **How to Know If Something Is Good:** Most hair products look pretty much the same when they're on the shelf, so the only way to tell if it's the right one for you is to try it. This can take some time and money. Start with something inexpensive and be prepared to try a few.
- **Don't Be Afraid to Ask:** The best thing to do is ask your barber what he uses. These guys have tried everything, and if they like something, you know it works. You can also ask a friend who has great hair what he uses. If there is a celebrity you think has especially great hair, Google them. There are plenty of articles out there where they, or their stylists, specifically talk about what products they use.

BARBERS VERSUS HAIRSTYLISTS

A man's barber is one of the most important people in his life. Whether you've gone to the same barber for years or have changed barbers are often as your clothes, the person who cuts your hair holds a lot of power. These relationships are built on trust, communication, and in many cases friendship. In some communities, the barbershop is the hub: an unofficial gathering place and social center of the neighborhood. Other guys don't want to say a word when they're in the barber's chair, and that's okay too.

Who cuts your hair is a personal choice, one that involves much more than literally getting your hair cut. When you look good, you feel good, and every barber or hairstylist wants their clients to feel amazing when they leave. Consider the person who cuts your hair to be one of your self-care Sherpas. Self-care might be about making yourself feel good, but it doesn't always have to fall on your own shoulders.

Choosing the person to cut your hair can be a big decision, which is why knowing the difference between barbers and hairstylists is important. There are obvious and subtle differences in what they do and what type of experience you'll have with each of them. Who you go to is up to you, but this is what you need to know in order to get the most out of it.

Barbers

Traditionally, barbers were trained to not only cut hair but also shave and trim beards. This is where the idea that barbers are for men and stylists are for women came from—women didn't need to get shaved. These days, though, the lines are blurred. Modern barbers still provide shaves and beard trims, but are mostly distinguished by the style of haircuts they do. They are typically trained to provide shorter, more traditional men's haircuts using clippers. The barber experience is usually simple. They don't often wash your hair before cutting it, they don't typically offer services like color, and they are typically pretty fast.

Why Go to One?
Barbers offer a no-fuss experience. Many shops offer walk-ins and an average appointment rarely exceeds half an hour. They also tend to be cheaper than a salon (though that's changing thanks to new high end barbershops). The biggest reason to go to one, though, is the type of haircut you're looking for. If you want something simple, like a crew cut or a fade, a barber is the best for you.

Why Not to Go to One
If your hair is longer or you want a haircut that requires more styling, consider a hairstylist instead. If you're looking for something beyond just a haircut, like color, skip the barbershop.

Hairstylists

What makes someone a hairstylist versus a barber comes down to training. Stylists have to get cosmetology licenses in order to work, which means they have to go to cosmetology school where they not only learn how to cut and style hair but also how to do things like color, perm, and give manicures. They typically use scissors

169

more often than clippers, another aspect of their different training. Hairstylists spend more time learning about cutting women's hair as well, which doesn't mean that they aren't able to cut men's hair, just that they approach it differently from a barber.

Why Go to One?

If you're looking for a longer cut or one that may require more styling, a hairstylist will be able to give that to you. Some say a cut from a stylist grows out better than one from a barber so you may not need to see them as often, but this depends on the cut you're getting. Stylists will typically wash your hair before cutting it. They'll also be able to do things a barber can't like color your hair or give you other treatments.

Why Not to Go to One

Stylists tend to be more expensive than barbers, and the appointments last longer. If you're looking for a quick appointment or a simple haircut like a buzz, stick to a barber.

How Much Is Too Much to Pay?

While the cost of a haircut is often a driving factor in where you choose to go, it shouldn't be the only factor. Don't just go for the cheapest option. You may not think people can tell when you have a cheap haircut, but they can. It comes down to attention to detail. Hair that is cut quickly and bluntly looks bad when it grows out, and if your neck isn't faded correctly or the edges are uneven, that's another sign your haircut was cheap.

This isn't to say that you have to spend hundreds of dollars on your hair every month. Do your research. Ask some friends with great hair where they go, read reviews of places near your home or job, or search *Instagram* for barbershops and salons where you live. Once you've found a few places you think look cool, check out their prices online. Choose the place with the highest price you are comfortable paying. Once you go, if you like the haircut, that's your new spot. If you don't like it, try the next one on your list.

How to Get a Haircut

Whether you've been going to the same place for years or are trying to find your new go-to, there are some tried-and-true rules to get the most out of the experience.

Get on a Schedule
You should be getting a haircut every four to six weeks. Nothing makes a haircut look sloppier than when your neck and sideburns are scraggly.

Use Pictures
If you're thinking of a new haircut or going to see a new barber, take pictures with you. Find a few shots of guys with the type of haircut you want and be prepared to articulate what you like about it.

Don't Use Words
Use your pictures instead. Trying to use barber terms you've heard other people use (like *fade* and *undercut*) is a recipe for miscommunication. Most barbers say their clients never use them properly.

Ask about Styling Up Front
When you're talking to your barber about your haircut, ask them about how to style it before they start. If you're not willing to put in the time to style it, you're not going to be happy with the result.

Remember: They're the Experts

If your barber says a certain cut won't look good on you, don't get frustrated. They're professionals and understand things about your hair and face shape that you might not. Talk to them openly and hear what they have to say.

A BRIEF HISTORY OF DAVID BECKHAM'S HAIR

There is not a man in the world who holds as much power over men's hair as David Beckham. It's rare to see a man who so obviously uses his hair as a tool for expression. He has had literally hundreds of hairstyles, all of them iconic. Here is a brief history.

- **2000: Buzz Cut:** Throughout the years, Beckham will go back to the buzz as a way to reset between styles.
- **2000: *Taxi Driver*:** Allegedly, he actually was inspired by Robert De Niro.
- **2003: Cornrows:** Let's just agree to forget this era.
- **2005: Fashion Mullet:** He also discovered headbands.
- **2014: Modern Pomp:** His short pompadour got millions of guys to learn the term "high and tight."
- **2018: Man Bun:** It's still a thing and we have Becks to thank.

SO, YOU'RE LOSING YOUR HAIR

We've spent a lot of time talking about how to take care of your hair, but the most important goal for lots of men is keeping it in the first place. Hair loss and thinning is the number one concern for nearly every guy, and chances are you're one of them.

It's not in your head either. Hair loss is an issue that impacts all men, regardless of age. The American Hair Loss Association says that two thirds of all men experience hair loss by the time they are thirty-five. As we get older, that number increases to 85 percent. Many experts say they typically start seeing patients complaining about hair loss in their early to mid-twenties, sometimes as young as their late teens.

Losing your hair can have negative effects on your self-esteem, personal relationships, sex life, and motivation. Many men see losing their hair as a sign of waning masculinity or loss of attractiveness. Self-care can be difficult when you're not happy with what's going on with your hair.

The reality is that most of it is genetic, as we'll get into, and you can't control whether it's going to happen to you. What you can do is treat it, the earlier the better. If you are convinced that you will lose your hair, like if everyone in your family is bald, take preemptive steps to slow the process. While you can't regrow hair that you've lost, you can retain it.

The first step is to see a professional who can advise you on the next plan of action. The next is to understand what's going on and experiment with treatments to find one that works for you. Be patient: Hair loss is a slow process and so is treating it. Most experts say that patients don't see a difference in their hair for three to six months after beginning treatment. When all else fails, there's always cutting your hair short and there's no shame in that either.

Why Does Hair Loss Happen?

The most common form of hair loss in men is androgenetic alopecia, commonly referred to as male pattern baldness (MPB). This form of hair loss is genetic; it's commonly thought that it comes from your mother's side (via X chromosomes), but growing research shows it can come from your father's side too. Spotting MPB is easy. A receding hairline, bald spot on the crown, and thinning on top of your head are all classic signs. It usually sticks to these areas, at least at first. Thanks to its genetic nature, there is not a lot you can do to prevent MPB, but you can control it.

While MPB is the most common, it's not the only kind of hair loss. Losing your hair can also be linked to internal diseases, poor diet, prescription medications, and even lifestyle. If you're noticing hair loss in areas other than the hairline or crown (like the sides or top of your head), this may be an indication that it's not MPB. Only an expert can tell for sure, so always consult a physician or hair loss expert before starting treatment.

How Does It Happen?

Scientists are not exactly sure, but they do know hair loss has to do with a male sex hormone called dihydrotestosterone (DHT) and an enzyme called 5-alpha-reductase, which helps to convert testosterone to DHT. The genes that cause MPB create an imbalance in this relationship and a higher amount of DHT in the scalp. When there is more DHT, certain hair follicles shrink and go dormant before dying off completely.

The life cycle of hair has three phases: the growth phase, the intermediate phase, and the shedding phase. In healthy hair, this cycle lasts around twenty-eight days, and hair that is shed is replaced with new growth. In scalps that have higher levels of DHT, the growth and intermediate phases are shortened, while the shedding phase is prolonged, which leads to thinning and loss.

Can It Be Cured?

It's been scientifically proven that once a hair follicle dies, it cannot be brought back to life. The good news is that it's next to impossible to tell if a hair follicle has died completely or just gone dormant. That means that even if you have large bald spots or think you're beyond help, you may still see some improvement from treatment. A doctor will be able to create a treatment plan specific to your needs, especially if your hair loss is not a result of MPB.

What to Do about It

The first thing you should do is see a doctor. Starting a treatment without medical advice could mean you're using the wrong one or you're starting one too early. Many treatments only show improvement for the duration of use, so starting them too early could mean you're locked in for the rest of your life. Most experts will create a customized routine for you out of some of these common treatments.

Over-the-Counter Products

Finasteride and minoxidil are the workhorses of the hair loss treatment industry. They regulate DHT both externally (minoxidil) and internally (finasteride). Recently, thanks to new generic options, these treatments are easily available in drugstores and online. They do not work if you stop taking them, however, and have some side effects, so be sure to consult your doctor first.

Scalp Care

Before beginning any hair loss treatment, make sure you're taking good care of your scalp. It will help promote an optimal environment for hair growth. Using a scalp scrub at least once a week to get rid of dead cells and product buildup is ideal, as is a scalp serum to help balance and hydrate the skin.

Natural Remedies

Thanks to the new holistic understanding of hair loss, more natural remedies are available than ever before. Botanicals like ginseng, ginkgo biloba, and holy basil are all said to help stimulate the scalp and promote hair growth and retention. Like any sort of supplement or drug, be sure to consult an expert before trying them yourself.

Technological Advances

The most promising new treatment is PRP, which stands for "platelet rich plasma," and is a substance extracted from the patient's own blood. This plasma is rich in growth factors, which, when injected into the scalp, have been clinically proven to help regrow hair. It's become the new gold standard in hair loss treatments.

LIFESTYLE MAKES A DIFFERENCE

It's not just about changing your products. Small changes in your lifestyle can have a big impact on your hair.

- **Sleep More:** If you're not getting enough high-quality sleep, the body's regenerative functions are impaired, which can lead to myriad health issues including hair loss. For more on the importance of sleep, turn to Part 2.
- **Eat Better:** The two ingredients integral to hair growth are protein and biotin. If you're not eating enough of either, your hair won't grow properly. Other ingredients like fatty acids, antioxidants, and zinc have also been shown to contribute to healthy hair growth.
- **Cut Stress:** Increased stress can force follicles into a dormant state or cause your immune system to attack them. If you're looking at hair loss holistically, decreasing stress is often one of the first goals.
- **Exercise (but Not Too Much):** Exercise is good for your health, but some studies have shown that excessive exercise has been linked to hair loss (temporarily). If you exercise a lot, make sure you're eating enough vitamins and proteins to account for it.

THE HAIR DOWN THERE

The word *manscaping*, invented by *Queer Eye for the Straight Guy* in the early 2000s, is totally cheesy, but male body hair grooming is nothing new. In ancient Egypt, for instance, body shaving was a way to deal with the oppressive desert heat. Today, body grooming is less of a necessity and more of a personal choice.

No one is required to manscape, but this is a book about self-care, and manscaping is a way to make yourself feel good. Many men don't like how certain body hair looks, especially as they get older and the same hormone that causes hair loss (DHT) makes hair on the body go wild. Seeing hair where it wasn't before can be jarring and many men take steps to get rid of it.

Other men want to keep it but make sure it doesn't grow too long. There are also other reasons to manscape: sports competitions, ingrown hair issues, excessive sweating, and helping things look a little bigger downstairs. Whatever your reason, there are plenty of ways to do it, even if you hate calling it "manscaping."

Types of Manscaping

Just like your hairstyle, how to groom your body comes down to your aesthetic choices.

Shaving

Just like a cleanly shaven face, a smooth body has certain perks. It's one of the quickest and most effective ways to completely get rid of hair you don't want but does take practice and upkeep.

Where to do it: Anywhere there is hair. It's best for places you can actually see (if you're going to do it yourself) and large areas like your arms, torso, and legs. Never try to do it yourself on areas like your back or butt that you can't see.

How to do it: If you've shaved your face, you can shave your body. Always do it in the shower or right afterward, where the warm water and steam help soften hair. Use a different razor on your body than you use on your face to help keep bacteria from cross-contaminating (certain bacteria like staph can spread easily).

Trimming

Trimming is the best way to control body hair without getting rid of it completely. It's also less harsh on your skin than shaving and many experts say it leads to fewer ingrown hairs and irritation, especially in sensitive areas like your groin. It's generally thought to be easier to do, so if you're a beginner, it may be a good way to dip your toe into manscaping without going full-shave.

Where to do it: Anywhere on your body, but especially in sensitive areas like your groin that are especially prone to irritation.

How to do it: Use a trimmer specifically designed for the body that comes with multiple length attachments. Start with the longest attachment and work your way shorter until you get the length you prefer. Never use the same trimmer on your body as on your face (that whole cross-contamination thing). Spread a towel or newspaper on the floor of your bathroom for easy cleanup and make sure you're standing in front of a mirror while you trim.

Waxing

Waxes, or other sticky substances, attach themselves to hair like glue and, when they're ripped off, take the full hair and root with them. Once waxed, the hair is completely gone until it regrows in the next cycle, which means a waxing job will last way longer than shaving. It's best for guys who don't want the regular upkeep of shaving or trimming.

Where to do it: Just like shaving and trimming, you can wax anywhere on the body that has hair, but since it usually involves another person to do it for you, it's ideal for places like your back or butt that are difficult to do yourself.

How to do it: Go to a waxing salon, period. There are plenty of at-home waxing kits you can buy, but if you've never been waxed before or are trying to do it in a sensitive area, leave it to the pros. It is quick, not nearly as painful as you'd expect, and you'll get better results.

Laser Hair Removal

If shaving your body is the Toyota Corolla of manscaping, laser hair removal is the Tesla. It's also permanent, so once you get rid of the hair, it never grows back. Depending on how much hair you want to remove and what color it is, it can take around eight sessions and can be expensive. For men who regularly manscape and want to completely get rid of hair for good, it's a small price to pay.

Where to do it: You can do it anywhere, but keep in mind that once you finish, that area will be hairless forever.

How to do it: Make an appointment with a professional. They'll be able to advise you on what to expect, how many sessions it will take to remove the hair, and how it will be done safely. Keep in mind that it can be expensive depending on where you go.

When to Seek Professional Help

Shaving and trimming can easily be done on your own, though some places now offer more customized services where they can contour your body hair like a haircut. Some men like this because how your body hair is cut can sometimes make your chest look more defined or draw attention to your abs. But most men can easily take care of general body grooming on their own.

Once you start considering waxing or laser hair removal, though, it's best left to professionals. You should always do research on online review sites or get personal recommendations before choosing a provider. If you're hoping to remove hair from hard-to-reach places like your back as well, those should be left to a professional to avoid cuts and uneven grooming.

GREAT MOMENTS IN GROOMING: THE 40-YEAR-OLD VIRGIN

When *The 40-Year-Old Virgin* came out in 2005, Steve Carell's screams could be heard echoing around the world. Professional waxers say that the scene is still referenced by male first-time clients to this day. Carell's screams of pain coupled with the grimaces of the onlookers have made waxing into something to be feared. In reality, a professional groomer would have likely trimmed Carell's chest rug before waxing to thin it out and make it less painful. They also would have gone quicker. The process of waxing is always much faster than you expect, which helps cut down on pain and makes the experience smoother.

Part 6

SPIRIT

So much of the wellness and self-care worlds have to do with things you can see or touch. There is also a lot of discussion about vibes, energies, emotional states, and levels of consciousness. It's confusing and it can even seem a little mystical. That's because self-care doesn't just benefit your physical body but your spiritual body too. This doesn't mean religion; it means the intangible energy inside all of us that connects us to the universe (however you conceptualize it). The tools that increase spiritual awareness can seem esoteric and impractical to skeptics, but even partial-believers can find surprising benefits.

As you get deeper into the self-care conversation, you might start rolling your eyes. That's okay! Self-care is a journey, not a destination. But you shouldn't discount the importance of spiritual health. Self-care practices that focus on more than just how your body feels are important. When reading about these more out-of-the-box tools, remember that they serve the same purpose as the other more common practices in this book: making yourself better. The only difference is that these aim to heal your mind and help you forge a meaningful connection with something outside of yourself. After all, we all need to feel like we're part of something.

NEW AGE IS NOW AGE

The term "New Age" was coined back in the seventies and eighties as a catchall category for weird stuff. Bookstores created New Age sections for their astrology books, record stores followed suit so they had a place to put Enya and Gregorian chant CDs, and every town eventually got a New Age store, which were basically incense emporiums. New Age was a descriptor for anything and anyone who was a little off the beaten path, at least when it came to spirituality.

Even back then none of these things were new. The whole concept of New Age depended on a "rediscovery" of centuries-old practices like yoga, meditation, and astrology. But in the face of eighties excess, New Age became something reserved for women with homemade earrings and men with gray ponytails.

These days, we call these same New Age concepts by another word: *wellness*. And no one is looking down on it, at least not in the same way. We can thank the Internet, the land of conspiracy theories and millennial angst, for the resurgence of concepts like astrology and tarot cards (this time in meme form). Truthfully, sociologists and other experts often say that in times of great stress, like political unrest or financial crisis, cultural interest in alternative forms of spirituality increases. It could also be that in today's screen-focused world, everyone is reaching for a little more connection. Basically, everyone wants to know there's more to their lives than the tweets they send.

As these "New Age" concepts become more mainstream, the fact of the matter is that alternative forms of healing and spirituality are tools. You can live a long and fulfilled life without any of them, but they can be useful in forging a stronger relationship with your inner self, the world around you, and the universe that holds us all. Many of these tools rely on the belief that there are unseen forces at work in the world around us, even in one's own body, and seeking to understand them can be helpful and healing.

Integrating one of these tools into your self-care practice is easy. It could be as simple as not skipping over the daily horoscope in the morning paper or having Reiki added on to your next massage. The best thing about the resurgence of these alternative forms of healing is that they are readily available. If you just open your eyes, you might be surprised.

Astrology

The ancient practice of astrology is more than just asking, "What's your sign?" at a bar. It's built on the idea that the planets in the solar system have an effect on people's lives similar to how the moon affects the ocean's tides. These invisible influences change as the planets move in their orbits through the twelve sections of the sky called the zodiac. Astrology is complex and hard to understand, which is why it's so mysterious. But paying attention to it, and learning from it, can help attribute meaning to some of the seemingly random parts of life.

How to Make It Self-Care: Astrology isn't a salve you can rub on your knee to make the pain immediately go away; it's more of a calming breeze in the background. You can't do anything to change the movements of the planets, but what's going on in the skies can hold answers to what's going on in your life. Paying attention to what's happening astrologically could provide answers to questions or reassurance that you're on the right path.

Reiki

Reiki is a Japanese form of energy healing where practitioners manipulate your energetic life force. When a person's life force is blocked, they can feel sluggish, stressed, and anxious—both physically and mentally. Reiki practitioners, or masters as they are called, can help get things moving and heal physically, mentally, and emotionally. Reiki masters use their hands and their own energetic flow to change yours.

How to Make It Self-Care: Many spas are now offering Reiki sessions, so if you see it on a spa menu, give it a try. You can also find a specific Reiki practitioner by doing online research and reading reviews. Reiki sessions are relaxing and stress reducing, but they aren't the same as a massage. Reiki masters are highly trained professionals, so in order to get Reiki, you have to see someone who knows what they're doing. Don't think you can DIY.

Tarot Cards

Most people think tarot cards tell your future, but they actually don't. The cards are a complex system of archetypal images that symbolize the life path of humanity. Tarot readers use these cards, and how they are arranged in a specific spread, to divine meaning from the images and offer a glimpse at what is happening in a person's life.

How to Make It Self-Care: Tarot is a tool for reflection and is best used to try to get answers to a question. If you're feeling confused, stuck, or stressed, using tarot to figure out what to do can be incredibly helpful. Learning to read tarot cards yourself takes practice because each card can have thousands of meanings. If you're interested in trying yourself, get a deck and a book for beginners and start drawing one card a day so you get a feel for what they are and what they mean. You could also find a reputable tarot reader in your area or even online (many popular tarot readers offer *Skype* or video chat readings).

Sound Baths

A form of meditation, sound baths use nonverbal sound to help you reach a deep meditative state. It's a similar idea to using a chant or mantra while meditating, but in this case, something else is making the sound. Sounds baths usually involve things like Tibetan singing bowls, gongs, chimes, or rhythmic drumming to create vibrations that affect your body. The thought is that these sounds and vibrations help you reach a deeper state of meditation and open your consciousness in ways you can't on your own.

How to Make It Self-Care: If you've ever played a certain song to relax, you get the idea of a sound bath. You can find recordings of singing bowls and gongs to play while you meditate, but finding a live sound bath can make a big difference in your experience. Look for meditation or yoga studios that offer sound baths, and give one a try.

Mediums

Mediums are people who have a specific connection to the spirit world and can communicate with forces on the other side. For skeptics, this can be a hard pill to swallow, but you don't have to completely believe in spirits to get something out of a medium. Most people seek them out because of a deep need to communicate with someone they have lost, but some just need guidance. Think of it as another form of therapy. Many mediums say everyone each has their own spirit guides who are constantly trying to communicate with us—the medium is simply the tool.

How to Make It Self-Care: Seeking out a medium takes some effort. They're few and far between, and not everyone who says they are a medium is legit. If you know someone who has been to one, ask for a referral. It's more likely that you don't, so head online. The good thing about mediums is that you don't usually have to be in the same place to meet with them, so look for ones who offer phone or video chat sessions. Enter your session with an open mind and heart and listen to what they have to say. What you get out of it depends on how well you listen.

IS THERE REALLY A NEW AGE?

The term "New Age" is attributed to a man named David Spangler, who believed that in 1970 the Earth had entered into a new cycle called the Age of Aquarius. The new cycle, or age, was characterized by an increase in spiritual energy that human beings could tap into and harness for their own spiritual development. Considered one of the architects of the New Age movement, Spangler believed that this age of heightened spiritual awareness would lead to drastic social change and set in motion a wave of renewed interest in things like yoga, meditation, astrology, and other more esoteric forms of spirituality. He created the New Age movement as we know it today. Some people believe that the new age is still to come, others believe we are smack-dab in the middle of it right now, and others are just happy there are yoga studios on every corner and meditation apps on their phones.

WHAT THE SMUDGE?

Maybe you've been in a yoga or meditation class when the teacher whipped out a bundle of leaves and lit them on fire. That teacher wasn't trying to burn down the room; it's called smudging, and it's used to help cleanse negative energy. In this context, the teacher is creating a neutral space that helps you focus on the practice you're about to do. Smudging can be used for more than that though.

Smudging, or the act of using the smoke of certain herbs and plants to dispel negative energy, has been used for thousands of years across many cultures. Certain smokes are thought to be able to change vibrations, manipulate energy, and even connect people with divinity. Think about how the Catholic Church uses incense in its services. Using scent and smoke to create sacred space is a form of smudging. Examples of smudging are found all over the world and, thanks to the wellness explosion, are more common than ever.

That's why now you see bundles of sage sold at fancy shops and sticks of palo santo being used as air fresheners in high-end bathrooms. As wellness and self-care practices become more popular, smudging is a common and easy way to change both your own energy and your surrounding environment.

Smudging is often referred to as "cleansing," a way to get rid of residual energy that could be bringing you down. Think of it this way: Negative energy is sticky, like grime on your mirror. Over time, without proper cleaning, it can build up and obscure the whole thing so you can't even see your reflection anymore. Smudging is like glass cleaner that will cut through it and bring the mirror back to its clear, normal self. There is even scientific backing to prove it. Certain "medicinal" smokes have been found to have positive effects on brain, lung, and skin functions, as well as have antiseptic properties in one's environment.

In self-care terms, smudging is helpful in many ways. It can help signal to your body and brain that you are about to start a particular self-care ritual like taking a bath or meditating. If you're stressed out, it can help calm you down; if you're feeling tired, it can help energize you; if you're feeling depressed, it can help lift your mood. It all comes down to the effects that negative energy can have on your psyche.

How to Know If You Have Negative Energy

Residual negative energy affects everyone in different ways. For some people, it makes them feel stressed, others sad or tired. Some people can't sleep well when there is too much negative energy floating around; others feel scattered and unable to focus. You may not even realize how negative energy is affecting your life until you've cleared it away.

One of the biggest sources of negative energy is other people. If someone you're close to is angry or upset, you can sometimes feel it without them saying anything at all. Think about times that you've had a big fight with someone and how those feelings can stick to you for days afterward, sometimes even years. Those are extreme situations, but negative energy can come from others even if they're not upset. How many times have you come home from a crowded party or busy day of meetings and felt exhausted? That's the energy of other people sticking to you. It's particularly common for people whose jobs depend on interacting with lots of people or shaking lots of hands. Everyone you meet has energy, and the more you encounter, the more it stays with you.

Negative energy is a bit of a misnomer since it doesn't always come from a bad place. It's just not *your* energy and it has a way of clogging things up if there is too much of it. Smudging is a way to reset your body and your surroundings to zero. It gets rid of buildup and blockages, like liquid plumber for your vibes.

Smudging Tools

When we talk about smudging, there are usually a few certain herbs or plants that are the most common. You could try using some oregano or thyme from your kitchen, but these will work much better.

Sage

Sage is the most common cleansing tool, specifically white sage. It's been used in many indigenous cultures for thousands of years to cleanse and purify space to get it ready for spiritual ritual. These days, it's still used for the same thing, but less mystically. Burning even a little bit can cleanse a space quickly and effectively. Some people find white sage too harsh, so investigate other gentler varieties if it's not your thing.

Palo Santo

This type of wood, whose name literally means "sacred wood," has been used to bless and consecrate sacred spaces for centuries in South America and beyond. Some say it doesn't have the same cleansing effect as sage but is still good for signaling intention and creating a relaxing environment.

Copal

Copal is a type of resin that, when burned, is thought to have an intense purification effect. Some say it also helps increase psychic awareness and facilitate higher consciousness. Copal originates from Mexico and other parts of Central and South America, where it is still used as a mosquito repellent.

Sweetgrass

Like sage, sweetgrass is common in Native American smudging rituals. However, these cultures believe that while sage has a cleansing and purifying quality, sweetgrass invites happiness and positive energy. The two are typically used together: first sage to get rid of negativity, followed by sweetgrass to facilitate positivity.

How to Smudge

Smudging is simple, literally just waving around a bit of smoke. To do it safely and effectively, though, you should follow these simple steps.

1. **Man the Exit:** Before you start, open the doors and windows of your space. Physically, this will help with airflow and allow the smoke to move around easier. Energetically, it helps to direct negative energy outside of your space and dissipate it away from you.
2. **Have a Backup Plan:** Always know where you're going to put out your smudge before you light it. Have a fireproof bowl or plate ready or, if you're particularly nervous, a bowl of water. Maybe keep it in the sink so you can easily extinguish it if there is a problem.
3. **Light It Up:** Now the main event: Light that sucker up. Smudging herbs are meant to smolder and produce lots of smoke, not a huge open flame. Once you've lit the herbs on

fire, let the flame die down until you see plumes of smoke instead or blow it out if it's not dying down on its own. Some smudges, like palo santo, may need to be relit throughout the process, so use a lighter and keep it in your pocket.

4. **Move with Purpose:** If you're cleansing a room, make sure to concentrate the smoke in every corner and spend extra time in front of windows or doors (where negative energy can come in). Some people say to walk around the room counterclockwise, but the most important thing is to try to get the smoke over as much surface as possible. The same goes for your body. Make sure to get the smoke over your hands, feet, and head—the places where energy enters your body most easily.

5. **Add Some Performance:** If you really want to go for the gusto, add a chant or sound to your cleansing. Some say that negative energy responds to sound, so things like clapping, humming, or yelling can help get rid of it faster. Even larger movements like jumping or dancing can help clear it out.

6. **Extinguish:** Once you feel you've sufficiently covered what you're trying to cleanse, extinguish the smudge in the container you set out before you started. Some say the best way is to grind it out, instead of using water, but whatever you use, make sure the fire is completely out before you put anything away.

WHEN TO SMUDGE

The general rule is that you should smudge whenever you need to get rid of negative, or excess, energy. What that means for you is that there really is no bad time. You can smudge:

- When you get home from work
- Before you meditate
- After a bad date
- After a dinner party
- After a road trip
- Before you take a bath
- After you have a fight with your family
- After your mother-in-law visits
- The first day of spring
- When you're on a deadline
- When you're having trouble sleeping
- Whenever you want to

GET OUTSIDE: WHAT NATURE CAN DO FOR YOUR MOOD

As humans, we seem to have been programmed to benefit from nature. How many times have you said, "I just need some fresh air"? Everyone knows the feeling of being outside, the sun on your face, the breeze in your hair, and the fresh air filling up your lungs. Great, right?

The problem is that not many people get it very often. Unless you're a park ranger, chances are you spend most of your time indoors (some studies have shown that the average person spends upwards of 93 percent of their time inside). It's a hazard of modern life that with most of everyone's life spent in front of a screen, they are lacking the time and desire to go outside just for the hell of it.

But getting outside could have real benefits for you, and science has proven it. It's known that plants emit oxygen as part of photosynthesis, which is why they're important to the health of the planet. As humans, higher oxygen content also has real benefits for how the body functions. It goes beyond that too; plants also produce phytoncides, which are essential oils that help trees and plants protect themselves against germs and infection. Phytoncides get into the air and are not only responsible for making the air in nature smell better, but they have been shown to have positive effects on the human immune system.

Studies have shown that spending time in nature, specifically doing a Japanese practice called *shinrin-yoku*, or "forest bathing," can have a positive impact on cardiovascular and respiratory health as well as increase the number of active immune cells in your body. The benefits go beyond the physical too. Psychological studies have also shown that forest bathing can decrease depression, anxiety, and confusion. It decreases the cortisol levels in your brain, which are attributed to stress, even for hours afterward.

These benefits can come from even a short time spent outside but ideally in a place like a forest or park where you're surrounded by trees and plants. And we're not talking going for a run or doing anything other than soaking it all in. Taking a good forest bath, and reaping the self-care benefits of *shinrin-yoku* in the process, takes very little effort.

How to Take a Forest Bath

Forest bathing is simple. Just follow these steps:

Give Yourself Time
When most people talk about forest bathing, they're talking about 2-hour sessions. If that amount of time sounds like too much for you to dedicate to a forest, don't stress. Figure out how much time you can spend, even 20 minutes or so, and commit to that.

Leave Your Phone Behind
It might sound scary to leave your best friend behind, but bringing your phone on a forest bath defeats the whole purpose. Leave it at home or in your car, along with any other technology you carry with you. Distraction is the kryptonite of any forest bath.

Don't Have a Goal
You probably do most things in your life because you're hoping to accomplish something. But forest bathing isn't about getting

somewhere—it's about the experience itself. If thinking of forest bathing as hiking helps you, so be it, but don't think of it as going to a specific place. Open yourself up to the experience instead of the destination.

Keep Your Senses Open

The point of forest bathing is to connect to nature. Take a look around you as you walk. Smell the air, touch the plants, listen to the sounds. A forest bath is about all your senses, and opening them up to what's around you makes all the difference.

Don't Rush

Since you're not going anywhere, what's your rush? Walk slowly and allow yourself to relax into the movement and surroundings. It might be uncomfortable at first, but letting yourself chill and enjoy nature will help you get more benefits in the long run.

Use the Time

Some people like to meditate or do yoga during a forest bath. That's cool too! If the idea of walking aimlessly stresses you out, find a place to sit down and take a moment. Using the quiet of nature to meditate can help you chill out even more.

Make It a Routine

Like anything worthwhile in life, getting the most out of forest bathing comes from consistency. One session feels great, but make it a habit. Try to go at least once a week, for as much time as you can spare, and increase the length or frequency if you can.

If You Don't Have a Forest

Forest bathing may sound great, but the problem most people face isn't desire to do it. It's access. Some studies have said that by the year 2050, 66 percent of the world's population will live in cities, which means that access to forests is not a reality many people have. If you're one of those people, don't worry! You can still get the benefits of forest bathing even if you're not in an actual forest. Head to a city park instead. Pick one that is large enough that you don't see roads or buildings when you're inside. Head for dense areas with larger trees if you can and try to find a quiet place to sit or walk. It's been shown that regular interaction with nature, even nature in the middle of a city, has the same benefits of walking in a natural forest. And if you don't have access to a park, create your own. Use your backyard or garden for the same effect. Spend time in a plant-filled area that you've created for yourself. If it's too small to walk around in, use it to meditate, do yoga, or just relax. It's not exactly the same as heading to the redwoods on a consistent basis, but you'll still get some of the benefits.

FOREST WALK WITH ME

If walking alone in the woods creeps you out, you're not alone! Many people have a hard time being by themselves, especially in places like a forest or a park. Luckily, there are groups for that. Forest bathing groups exist in all areas of the country (and the world), and a good place to look for them is the Internet. Look for meetups in your area (many of them are free) or private groups that go on regular forest bathing excursions. There are also trained guides who regularly hold forest bathing excursions on a private and public basis. Check out the Association of Nature and Forest Therapy Guides and Programs to find trained guides in your area.

A NOTE ON EARTHING

The practice of earthing is simple: It's literally standing out-side barefoot. The idea is that by removing shoes and any-thing else that stands between your feet and the earth, you are able to form a more direct connection to nature. It is said to have a grounding effect on your body's energy, the same way electrical circuits are usually grounded. While earthing is not required during a forest bath, it can add to its benefits. Even standing barefoot in your yard for a few minutes a day can have grounding and de-stressing benefits. Wherever you plan to earth, always check the ground before taking off your shoes. Make sure there aren't any sharp objects or things that could hurt your feet. Look for areas of soft grass or dirt so your feet sink into the earth, and if you walk around, do it carefully.

WTF IS UP WITH CRYSTALS?

You may not realize that crystals are all around you. Sure, you've seen them in stores being sold as cool decorative objects, dotting the shelves at health food cafes, and popping up around yoga studios and meditation classes. You have even seen them in your friends' homes and sitting on your coworkers' desks and definitely all over *Instagram*. But crystals are also in your cell phone, your TV, your computer, and probably your watch. That's because crystals are not just cool-looking chunks of rock. They are minerals with unique molecular structures, some of which have the ability to conduct electricity, and all of which have majorly high vibrations.

Using crystals for their vibrations is nothing new. Every civilization ever recorded has used crystals in some way. In ancient times, these minerals were identified for their unique energies and used in spiritual and healing rituals. They have the ability to absorb and conduct energy (all kinds, not just electricity) and have always been used as valuable spiritual conduits. In fact, certain crystals are said to have been programmed with the knowledge of previous lost civilizations, like a sort of prehistoric USB drive. Plus, you know, they look cool.

Modern interest in crystals has spiked and not just for their technological prowess. Like most things in this book, you can thank the wellness and self-care movements for the cultural refascination with crystals. Their power never waned, but people's interest did. Now you can find entire *Instagram* accounts dedicated to them, thousands of books being sold on how to use them, and even skincare products claiming to harness their power.

What does this mean for you? Well, it means that understanding crystals and how to use them could take your self-care practice to the next level. They're so powerful that this entire book could be about crystals, but in practice it's really pretty simple. Here's how to get started.

The Best Crystals for Dudes

The first step in using crystals is starting to understand the thousands of varieties and what each does. These are some of the most common and easiest to use.

Clear Quartz

Quartz is the MVP of the crystal world, particularly the clear variety. It's probably what pops into your mind when you think "crystal" anyway: a translucent pointy thing that looks like glass. Any exploration of crystals has to begin with clear quartz because it's the most versatile. It's like a blank sheet of paper and is able to be programmed to whatever intention you want. If you're not sure what kind of crystal you need to use for something, grab a quartz. It can also amplify the vibrations of other crystals, like a subwoofer on your stereo.

Rose Quartz

You can tell rose quartz by its pink color, which also gives a clue to what it's used for: love. It's good at inviting new relationships, making existing ones stronger, and even creating a more loving and supportive relationship with yourself (self-love is important too). It also has a calming and soothing effect. Rose quartz wants to harmonize situations and bring them into balance.

Amethyst

You've seen this crystal used a lot in jewelry and decorative objects because of its beautiful deep purple color, but it's more than just cool to look at. It's a protective stone, which helps dispel negative energy like a force field. It's also said to have spiritual properties and can help you reach a higher state of consciousness and increase psychic abilities.

Selenite

Unlike most crystals, selenite is so delicate that it can't get wet. It's made up almost entirely of salt, which is why it's ideal for cleansing a space. Selenite kept in your house or your office will soak up negative vibes like a sponge and keep your energy fields clear and positive. It's also self-cleansing, meaning it gets rid of negative energy by itself instead of storing it.

Citrine

Citrine's golden orange or yellow color is like a ray of sunshine, which is why it's always been associated with the power of the sun. It invites positivity, creativity, and happiness. Think of it as the "Most Likely to Succeed" of the crystal world; citrine is always excited and ambitious. It's good for manifesting hopes and dreams and inviting prosperity. Keep it in the sunlight for extra power.

Black Tourmaline

Dark crystals are like little factories; they absorb negative energy and convert it into positivity. Keep a chunk of black tourmaline with you and it will help absorb negativity you encounter on a daily basis. Keep some at your desk to stay chill in the face of a mean boss, or grab some right after a fight with your significant other. Keep in mind that any negative energy–sucking crystal like this needs to be cleansed regularly to help get rid of built-up badness.

Pyrite

You may know it as "fool's gold" because it looks like gold, but isn't. However, it is still a powerful wealth manifester, especially if you have your own business. Keeping it near a cash register or in your wallet will help attract wealth. It's also grounding and heart-opening, which can be helpful for entrepreneurs.

How to Use a Crystal

Once you figure out what crystal you need, the next thing to do is actually use it. Here's how:

Cleanse It

Before using your crystal, especially the first time, you want to cleanse it to get rid of any energetic leftovers (like from other people who have touched it). First, sprinkle it with salt water (unless it's selenite) and make sure you cover the whole thing. Next, light up some sage or other smudging herb and pass the crystal through the smoke a few times. Make sure to turn it so the smoke covers the entire crystal.

Program It

You've chosen a certain crystal for a specific reason, but it's still dormant until you activate it. Think about why you've chosen it and what you hope to accomplish. Hold the crystal in your hands and send the mental picture you have into the crystal like you're uploading a file. You could say what you want out loud in words or simply visualize your desired result. If it helps, picture dragging a file (your intention) into a USB drive (the crystal).

Harness It

Programming your crystal is the hard part. Harnessing it is easy. Once it's been linked to your intention, you can use it in a variety of ways. You could meditate with the crystal in your hands or on the ground in front of you. You could put it in the water while you're taking a bath (water can amplify vibrations). You could keep it on your desk at work or in your bag. You can put it in a special place, like next to your bed or on the fireplace mantel, where you can see it regularly. No matter how you use it, make sure you come in contact with it regularly.

Repeat It

Depending on your intention, and how often the crystal comes in contact with other energies, you need to reprogram it regularly. Always re-cleanse it before setting a new intention as a way to start with a clean slate each time and make sure there isn't a buildup of energy. You could use the same intention each time you program or switch it up depending on how you're feeling.

INFINITY STONES IRL

A decade of Marvel movies revolved around one premise: a bunch of crystals that were so powerful they could end the universe. When you really think about it, *Avengers: Infinity War* and *Avengers: Endgame* were basically about a bunch of dudes obsessed with rocks. Sure, the hunk of clear quartz you bought off of *Amazon* isn't going to stop time, but think about crystals as your own Infinity Stones. They have power of their own that might not turn you into an Asgardian hero or iron-clad man-robot, but they can still make major things happen if you use them right. Just keep them away from Thanos.

GRATITUDE IN THE SOCIAL MEDIA AGE

Everyone's been there: scrolling through social media and finding picture after picture of amazing vacations, delicious meals, happy relationships, fancy cars, fit bodies, fun parties, etc. After a while, it can be dizzying. "How are all of my friends' lives perfect?" you ask yourself as you sit on your couch eating a microwaved dinner. It's hard not to compare yourself and your life to what you see on social media, especially the more you see it.

We all know that what's presented on social media is not always reality, but that doesn't make it easier to stomach. It's easy to remind yourself that you're seeing what people want you to see, but it's even easier to start feeling like your life doesn't measure up. While your friends are on vacation, you're stuck at work; while one of your friends is test driving a Maserati, you're on the bus; while one of the fitstagrammers you follow is checking his eight-pack abs in a mirror, you haven't been to the gym in weeks.

Social media can have a real effect on your self-esteem in the present and the future. Right now, it makes you jealous that you don't have what other people do. Down the road, it can warp your perception of what is realistic, achievable, and meaningful.

One of the best ways to keep these feelings in check is to, of course, put down the phone. But that can only go so far. As self-care tools go, creating a gratitude practice can help you keep things in perspective, build your self-esteem, and maintain a positive outlook, even when your friends post vacation selfies for weeks after they come back.

What Is Gratitude?

Put simply, the practice of gratitude is being grateful. It sounds simple, like something you probably already do around the Thanksgiving table, but in practice it's difficult. Humans are programmed to want what we don't have. It's what keeps us striving for that next raise, that bigger house, those bigger biceps. It's human nature. Gratitude, however, reminds you to appreciate what you have right now and invites you to find happiness in what you might be overlooking on a daily basis.

Why Does It Help?

Those who practice gratitude say that they have less stress, sleep better, have lower anxiety, and generally have a more positive and happy outlook on life. There are actually studies to back this up too. Some studies have shown that while gratitude practice helps people become happier in the moment, it also helps them stay happier in the long term (one study showed that something as simple as writing a thank-you note kept subjects happier for a month afterward).

Think of the practice of gratitude as maintaining the mortar on a brick wall. Over time, erosion breaks down the mortar between the bricks. In this scenario, the bricks are your mental health and erosion is negative emotions. Without proper maintenance, the mortar crumbles away leaving the wall unstable and weak. But by maintaining the mortar, the wall stays strong for years. Gratitude works the same way. Consistent practice keeps your emotions strong, your outlook positive, and your life happier.

How to Build a Gratitude Practice

It's easy to make gratitude part of your daily self-care practice. It just takes a little commitment.

Start with a List

The beginning of any gratitude practice starts with identifying what you're grateful for in your life. This should come in the form of a list, especially the first time you do it. You want to be able to identify everything that is good in your life and everything that makes you happy. Be thorough and take time to really think about it.

Write It Down

Instead of making your list in your head, actually put pen to paper. This helps clarify your thoughts and also allows you to go back and read it later. Some people keep gratitude journals specifically for this purpose. Having a record and going back to read it often will not only help keep gratitude at the front of your mind but can show you how your mindset changes over time.

Be Specific

The point of gratitude is to adjust your thinking so you start focusing on new and positive things instead of negative thoughts. It's fine if you start out writing down things like "I'm thankful I have food to eat," but each day try to get more specific. The more specific you can be in your gratitude practice, the more you will be able to see all the things you are grateful for in your life.

Be Consistent

Like anything, the key to a healthy gratitude practice is consistency. Find time to do a little bit every day. It takes around sixty-six days to form a habit, so try to force yourself to create one out of gratitude. If you use a gratitude journal, use the same one every day. Find a way to integrate gratitude into your daily routine, like journaling while your coffee is brewing in the morning.

Keep It Fresh

Try not to repeat yourself every day. After a while, you'll see patterns, and if you keep things too general, you may fall into the trap of writing down the same thing every day. Try to find a few new things each day to be grateful for. It can be as simple as a change in weather or having something different for breakfast.

Find Time Throughout the Day

When you first start a gratitude practice, dedicating the same time every day can be helpful. But as you get further, try to find new pockets of time throughout the day to practice gratitude. Keeping gratitude at the forefront of your mind will help you maintain a positive attitude in the face of stress. Journal or think about your gratitude during your lunch break, during your commute, or on your way to dinner after work to keep the good vibes flowing.

Be Flexible

Positive thinking is at the core of any gratitude practice, so be careful to not pressure yourself and make it start feeling like a chore. If you are feeling down and having a hard time coming up with things to be thankful for, don't press it; be compassionate to yourself and give yourself permission to try again tomorrow.

Start Giving

Many people who practice gratitude say that it not only helps them have more compassion for themselves, but also for others. To take your gratitude practice to the next level, start paying it forward. Carry some change to give to needy people on the street instead of walking by; help an elderly person get off the bus instead of grumbling behind them; offer a homeless person your leftover lunch instead of throwing it out.

WHEN *INSTAGRAM* IS GETTING YOU DOWN

Gratitude can be a big help in cutting through the visual clutter of *Instagram*. It can help remind you that what you have in your life is exactly what you need. But sometimes we need a little extra help. Here's what to do if *Instagram* is getting you down.

1. **Limit your time.** Use your phone's screen time tracker to limit the time you can access *Instagram* per day.
2. **Unfollow people who make you feel bad about yourself.** You may be following all those fitstagrammers for workout motivation, but they can start making you feel bad about your body.
3. **Mute your friends when they're on vacation.** Ask to see their vacation photos when they come home instead.
4. **Remember, influencers are not your friends.** They're trying to sell you things, including a cool lifestyle, and what they present on social media is not reality.

HOW TO BE AN EXTROVERT

In the conversations around self-care, even in this book, there is a lot of focus on things you do by yourself. That's by design: The act of self-care is literally taking care of yourself. It's a way to get in touch with your body, understand your own needs, and show your physical and emotional bodies that you value them. We've already established why this is important (everything from decreasing stress, helping you live longer, and, yes, even looking better).

But so much focus on the individual leaves behind something equally important: your relationships with other people. Relationships are important for human development and long-term health. Studies have shown that individuals with strong personal relationships manage stress better, are generally healthier, and may even live longer. Conversely, people with few or no meaningful relationships in their lives are at a higher risk for depression, heart disease, and obesity among other issues.

These issues seem to be getting worse as more and more people spend time behind screens instead of interacting with others face to face. Younger generations find it hard to form meaningful connections offline, and some experts say social anxiety disorders are on the rise. One of the reasons could be fear. The anonymity afforded by the Internet is like a safety blanket, where you don't have to risk the possibility of rejection or awkwardness.

In any self-care conversation, the value of personal relationships should not be discounted. The point of self-care is to create a meaningful and healthy life for yourself, and that's nearly impossible if you are always by yourself. Like anything, it's always about balance. Even the most extroverted person needs time alone to recharge and take care of themselves. On the flipside, introverts need meaningful personal interaction in order to be happy. No matter where you fall in the spectrum, start conceptualizing a well-rounded idea of self-care. It's not just how many baths you take but how everything in your life benefits you and those around you.

Can You Teach Yourself to Be More Outgoing?

To be clear, there is nothing wrong with being an introvert. Studies have shown that introverts make up anywhere from 30–50 percent of the population. But being an introvert is not the same as being a recluse. Introverts still need personal relationships. They just favor fewer, more meaningful ones.

If you have a hard time interacting with people, or forming relationships with others, there are ways that you can teach yourself to be more outgoing. Think of it as public self-care.

Listen

Many experts say that true introverts are not always great listeners. Instead they spend time in their own heads; they're worried about whether they said something wrong or seem awkward to the other person. Instead, when talking to another person, make a conscious effort to actually listen to what they are saying. Ask questions about what they are saying that will keep them talking. Focus entirely on what they're saying, and try to block out negative thoughts you might be having.

Visualize

If social settings give you anxiety, visualization exercises can be helpful. Before going into a meeting or a party, close your eyes and visualize yourself smiling, laughing, and interacting with everyone. Spend time really developing the picture, so you have a clear image of how well you're doing talking to others. These visualizations can help push fear and anxiety aside and open your mind to new interactions.

Give Yourself Permission to Fail

No one is good at something the first time they do it. If you don't do as well as you'd hoped in a conversation or social setting, don't let it discourage you. Try again next time. Remember that not everyone you meet will become your best friend and it's okay if you meet someone you don't particularly like (or they don't seem to like you). Forming relationships takes time.

Take "No" Out of Your Vocabulary

For introverts, the gut reaction to most invitations is "no." Stop saying it. Accepting all types of invitations opens up new experiences, and if you don't try it, you may not find out you like it. An invitation could be to a post-work coffee with a new coworker, to the party of an acquaintance you haven't seen in years, or even just into a conversation with your local barista.

Accept Yourself

Having compassion for yourself is most important, and accepting who you are is part of that. If you're introverted by nature, it doesn't mean you have to suddenly become the life of the party. Opening yourself up to new people and new experiences doesn't mean you have to completely change your life. Look for a balance you feel comfortable with.

How to Share Self-Care

Self-care is a perfect way to connect with yourself and your body, but it can also be a great way to connect with others. Including people in self-care practices is easy and can open your mind as well as theirs.

Invite Someone

If you're heading somewhere like a spa or meditation class, invite a friend to come along with you. Think about someone who you know is interested or who you think could benefit from the experience and reach out. They won't be able to say yes if you don't ask.

Participate in Group Activities

Instead of always practicing self-care by yourself at home, start taking it public. Look for group classes or meetups where people who are interested in the same things as you come together. It could be a workout class, a forest bathing group, or a book club. Use message boards or online review sites to find groups if you don't know anyone with your same interests.

Use Social Media

Social media can be a valuable tool in community building. If you don't know anyone IRL who's into meditation, for instance, start following meditation accounts and interact with them. Look for message boards where other people talk about shared interests. Knowing that there are other people to talk to about self-care can make a big difference.

Talk about It

Talking about your self-care practices in real life can be an important first step in forging relationships. You may not know one of your friends is also into self-care if you never talk about it, right? Don't wait for other people to bring it up. Start the conversation, and chances are your friends or family will want to know more and may even ask you to do it with them.

Open Your Mind

As you form more meaningful relationships with others around self-care, you may encounter other practices you've never thought of yourself. Don't discount them! Keep an open mind and try new things when others invite you. You may find something you like even more than what you're already doing!

ALONE TIME TIPS FOR EXTROVERTS

Even the most outgoing extrovert needs some alone time now and then. Just like meaningful relationships are important for your health, so is time spent alone. If you have a hard time being by yourself, try these tips.

- **Turn off your phone.** Constant text alerts and calendar invites can take you out of the present. Keep your phone off for a set period of time to allow you to not get distracted.
- **Schedule alone time.** Find a period of time, maybe about an hour, each week and block it into your schedule. This could be the time you take a self-care-focused bath or read a book you've been meaning to pick up.
- **Decline an invitation.** Instead of saying yes to everything, pick one thing to politely decline each week. Overpacked schedules lead to stress.

Part 7

SPACE

No matter how much time you spend there, your home is an important part of your life. It should reflect your taste and style, sure, but it's even more important that it's a place you feel comfortable. So many of the self-care tools and techniques discussed in this book can be done at home (which is an important part of a healthy self-care routine), but if your home isn't a place you want to be, it can be hard to chill out enough to focus on self-care. It should never be hard to relax in your own home, but when it is, it's next to impossible to form an effective self-care routine.

Everyone would love to live in a mansion with all sorts of space to dedicate to self-care. A private gym, maybe, or a dedicated meditation room sounds great, but they're not really necessary to create an effective and constructive self-care routine. For many people, that's not realistic. The good news is that it doesn't matter! Any home can be optimized for self-care regardless of how big it is. With minimal effort, a few strategic changes, and maybe a few houseplants or scented candles, your house can become a spa-level self-care palace.

HOW TO TAKE YOUR HOME FROM MAN CAVE TO SELF-CARE PALACE

All it takes to optimize your home for self-care is a little rethinking. Creating multiuse spaces is a good way to start. If you're tight on space, rethink how the space is set up and conceptualize all the things you can do (a reading nook can double as a meditation and yoga area, for instance). Start organizing your home around your self-care routine instead of the other way around.

Secondly, keep it clean. You don't have to watch Marie Kondo on *Netflix* to know that clutter leads to stress. Creating a space you feel comfortable in is not a license to hoard. Psychologically, clutter is like a sponge for negative energy; physically, it can block airflow and impair breathing.

Creating a welcoming and positive space is a personal experience. Surround yourself with things that make you happy and invite relaxation. Remember: Your home is where you should be able to rest and recharge. To help make it the best it can be, go room by room and follow these steps.

Living Room

Start with the room you spend most of your time in. Chances are it's the living room.

Seating Is Fundamental

The most important part of the living room is the seating, and for most people seating revolves around the couch. Choose a couch that's proportionate to the room and doesn't overwhelm it. That may mean going smaller than you want, but if that's the case, choose a couple accent chairs too. Make sure they look good together and are all equally comfortable.

Don't Make the TV the Focal Point

Let's face it: You probably spend most of your time at home in front of the TV. Instead of organizing the room around the TV, mount it up on the wall out of the way or put it in a corner. You want to create a relaxing vibe for yourself and a space where conversation with guests flows easily, without the TV looming over you.

Set the Lighting

Switch out harsh overhead lighting for a softer fixture with multiple bulbs to help spread the light across the room. Invest in a few accent lamps too so you aren't always dependent on the overhead fixture. An easy upgrade for every room, like if you rent your apartment and can't switch fixtures, is to install dimmers on the light switches. It helps manage light to your exact tastes.

Rugs, Not Carpet

Instead of installing wall-to-wall carpet, which can mask sounds but hold on to allergens, go for hardwood floors. Not only are they easier to clean but they help facilitate better airflow throughout the space. Find a cool accent rug (or a few) that you like and place them around the room, like under the coffee table or chairs, to help protect the floor and muffle sound.

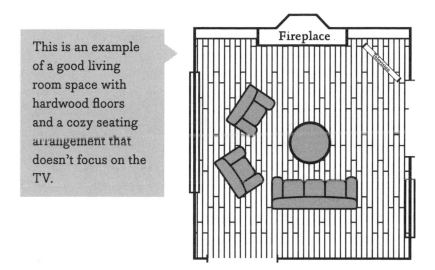

This is an example of a good living room space with hardwood floors and a cozy seating arrangement that doesn't focus on the TV.

Get Some Real Art

Nothing makes a room look instantly homier than some art, but we're not talking movie posters or record sleeves. Art doesn't have to be expensive: You can find a cool photo online and have a high-quality printout made, get a cool piece from a rummage sale, or find inexpensive original prints on websites like *Etsy*. Use an online framing service to have it framed on the cheap.

Kitchen

Creating a kitchen you actually want to be in could mean you spend more time cooking for yourself.

Organize Your Stuff

Keeping your food and tools organized not only makes it easier to find what you need but also makes your kitchen easier to clean.

Invest in a spice rack so you're not always digging through cabinets. Put your loose items (like flour or nuts) in clear glass containers that look good and make it easy to see what's inside.

Keep the Fridge Clean

A dirty fridge not only looks terrible but it can also keep your food from lasting as long. Wipe down the shelves and drawers regularly and make sure you throw out old or expired food quickly and often. Keep an open box of baking soda on one of the shelves to help soak up odors. And every time you clean the inside, remember to wipe down the outside too.

Back to Basics

Cooking at home is great for your wallet and your self-care, but for many people cooking can be stressful. Make it easier on yourself and invest in basic kitchen tools like pots and pans, spatulas, knives, and cutting boards. Having the right tools around will make cooking easier and quicker. If you're not sure what you need, look for a precurated kitchen kit with all the basics included, and if you don't know how to use them, look up some videos on *YouTube* or take a knife skills class.

Upgrade Your Dish Soap

Simply changing the scent of your dish soap can completely change how you feel about being in your kitchen. Citrus scents are energizing and invigorating, and floral scents like lavender are calming. It may make washing dishes less terrible, and after you're done, the smell will linger in the kitchen (in a good way).

The Table Factor

Even if you only have a little bit of space, putting a small table and a few chairs in your kitchen completely changes the vibe. It helps to have a place to eat that's not your couch or in front of the

TV, and it also invites other people into the room while you're cooking. Cooking can sometimes feel isolating, but if there is someone else there, it completely changes the experience.

Even if your kitchen is small like this galley version, a table makes it feel more homey.

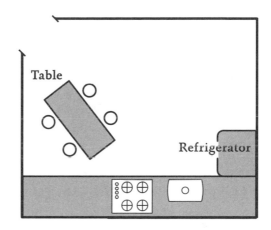

Bedroom

It's said that the average person spends one third of their life sleeping. Make it easier by making sure your bedroom is primed for sleep.

Get More (or Better) Pillows

Having more than one pillow on your bed not only makes it better when you're not the only one in it, but it can mean you have a more restful sleep. Find a few different pillows of different softness so you can find the right combination for your best sleep. Try stacking pillows or switching them up till you find the one that gives you the best sleep.

Invest in Sheets

Quality sheets can mean all the difference in how well you sleep. When buying sheets, don't get hung up on the thread count.

Look at the material first (linen sheets tend to be the most breathable, and flannel sheets will keep you warm when it's cold outside) before the thread count. Always feel sheets before you buy them, or take advantage of trial offers, so you can make sure the texture is exactly how you want it. And always get the matching pillowcases.

You Need a Table

No matter how much space you have in your bedroom, try to fit in a bedside table. Keeping things like your alarm clock or a book accessible will help create a relaxing environment and facilitate your bedtime routine (turn back to Part 2 for a refresher on that).

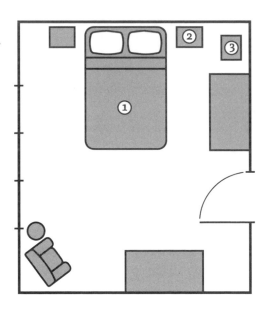

This bedroom layout is ideal. The bed (1) does not have either side against a wall and does not angle your feet toward the door (which is the "death position" in feng shui). It also has a nightstand (2) on either side of the bed and a hamper (3) in the corner for containing dirty clothes.

Put Your Clothes Away

Nothing clutters up a bedroom faster than clothes, so invest in a hamper and use it. Keep it in a corner or in the closet and remember to always put dirty clothes inside instead of on the floor or bed. Dirty clothes hold on to odors and impede airflow inside your bedroom, a place where the air quality is of utmost importance.

Double Blind

Remember that light is important for sleep and you want to be able to get enough natural light in your bedroom. Invest in some blinds, which can help filter light in and out, as well as curtains to block out light when you have trouble sleeping.

TO KONDO OR NOT TO KONDO

Ever since Japanese lifestyle guru Marie Kondo came out with her bestselling book *The Life-Changing Magic of Tidying Up* (and subsequent TV series), more people have come to understand the power their surroundings have on their mood and mental state. Her main point? If something in your home doesn't "spark joy," you need to get rid of it. It sounds straightforward, but it's a lot harder to do than it sounds. It doesn't necessarily mean it's a great way to organize your life. For some people, lots of stuff sparks joy; for others, not much. Take a page from her book, but don't treat it as gospel. The most important part of your home is that you feel comfortable. So if you like stuff, that's cool. If you're a minimalist, more power to you.

FENG SHUI THE RIGHT WAY

Your body has specific energy fields that, when blocked, can have real effects on your physical and mental well-being. According to the ancient Chinese art of feng shui, the same can be said of your home.

In feng shui, it is believed that the spaces you inhabit contain energy as well (called *chi*), and by facilitating the flow in certain ways, you can literally change the way your house makes you feel. Think about it: You may have certain rooms in your house that you feel more comfortable in than others. You might not be able to put your finger on why, but you know it's true. You're picking up on the energy currents that are swirling around you, and when they are positive you feel better.

Feng shui has been used for thousands of years, often to conceptualize how to build temples and other religious structures but also in commercial and residential building as well. It's thought that creating a building with good feng shui from the beginning invites positivity, prosperity, and longer lives to the occupants. You may not have a lot of control over how your house or apartment was built, but that's okay. Making a few changes to how you've set things up inside can change the feng shui too.

Using feng shui to create a more relaxing, comforting environment can make your self-care routine easier. Just like you've decorated your home to create a place where you feel comfortable, using these tips to optimize energy flow can take your self-care to the next level.

How to Start

In order to properly feng shui your home, you first need to understand the whole picture.

Focus on the Positive

Think about the rooms you feel most comfortable in and try to identify why that is. Maybe you have positive memories in a specific room, or the color of the walls speaks to you. Maybe you have mementoes or plants in your favorite room but not in the others. Try to identify a few things you like best about your favorite rooms so you can understand what you respond to on a deeper level.

Don't Forget Anything

No matter how big your house or apartment, start by going through every space. Look in every closet and don't leave out any room. You might not think that the laundry room you never go in or the storage room behind the kitchen matters, but in feng shui, the house is viewed as one entity, just like a human body.

Pay Attention to Doors and Windows

One of the biggest parts of feng shui is understanding how energy enters and leaves your house. Start with the front door and look to see what it opens into. If there are stairs directly in front of it, for instance, energy might swoop upstairs instead of circulating through the first floor. Move on to the internal doors to see if you can identify circuits or blockages. Look at the windows too and see if they open into the air or if they're blocked by anything from the outside.

Get Rid of Clutter

Before starting any feng shui makeover, you need to get rid of clutter. Not only can it physically impede airflow and keep dirt and dust inside, but it also blocks energy. Think of clutter as a clog in an artery: The more there is, the harder everything has to work to get around it. You don't have to get rid of everything, but try to pare down what you can.

Optimize the Flow

Once you've done an initial feng shui sweep of your home, start with a few small adjustments that can make a big difference.

Keep the Bathroom Door Closed

In feng shui, water symbolizes wealth, and the bathroom is the place where water leaves your house. Keeping the bathroom doors closed (and the toilet seats down) is said to prevent wealth from being swept away with the water.

Leave Room on Both Sides of Your Bed

If only one side of your bed is open, like if it's pushed up against a wall, then you're shutting yourself off to the possibility of love. Even if you're not in a relationship, make sure both sides of the bed are accessible as a signal to the universe that you are inviting companionship.

Get Some Mirrors

In feng shui, mirrors are useful tools at diffusing and directing energy. If you think a room is stagnant, put a mirror on the wall to keep things moving. Mirrors also do well at the end of hallways so energy doesn't get caught in a loop. Just keep mirrors out of the bedroom because they're thought to stir up energy and make it hard to sleep.

Isolate Electronics

According to feng shui, electronics are believed to emit energy that disrupts the natural flow of chi. This is especially important in the bedroom, where they can alter sleep patterns, so keep electronics like TVs and computers away from the bedroom when you can. Doing away with them from your home entirely is impractical, but try to keep them relegated to certain rooms.

Face Your Furniture Toward the Door

In each room, try to face furniture toward the door. Not only will this make the space look more inviting and facilitate better airflow, but feng shui believes that it creates a positive energy flow. It also helps with security too since you'll always be able to see when someone enters a room. The exception to this rule is your bed. The foot of the bed should never face a door that enters into the room (this is called the death position and is bad news).

Pay Attention to Colors

In design and in feng shui, colors are important. It's advised to stay away from bright colors, which can create an energetic frenzy. Instead, choose soothing colors for the walls and fabrics of a room. This doesn't necessarily mean muted, but consider each space and what mood you evoke. You can even go deep to figure out what element is associated with your birth date in feng shui and use colors to balance it.

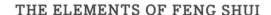

THE ELEMENTS OF FENG SHUI

Feng shui uses five elements—earth, air, fire, water, and metal—to create balance. When one or more of these elements is out of balance, it's believed to invite in negative energy. Each element has associations, like color, scents, sounds, and textures, but you don't have to do much research to figure them out. For instance, red is associated with fire, so if you have a red couch, balance it out with something blue in the space (like a rug or wall color) so it doesn't lean too far into fire. Lots of windows in a room invite light and the air element, so ground the room with plants or other earth-element symbols. Like most other things, it's all about balance.

HOW TO BUILD A BETTER BATHROOM

"Why is there an entire section devoted to the bathroom?" you might be asking yourself. Because let's get real: When it comes to actually doing most of the things discussed in this book, you'll be doing them in the bathroom. Your bathroom is like self-care ground zero. Unless you're taking a bath in your kitchen sink or washing your face outside with the hose, your self-care routine means spending time in the bathroom.

It's something you should want to do, but if your bathroom itself isn't a place you want to be, you're much less likely to take time for self-care. You already have enough reasons to *not* take care of yourself, but switching your thinking might mean switching up how you feel about your environment.

The easiest way to do this is to give your bathroom a self-care-focused makeover. That doesn't mean taking a sledgehammer to the walls like you're someone on HGTV. It means looking at your bathroom in a new way. Instead of thinking of it as a place you go when you need to or a place you want to get in and out of as quickly as possible, start thinking of the bathroom as a refuge. You might laugh when you see people on *House Hunters* say they want their bathroom to have a "spa atmosphere," but they're on to something. In the world of self-care, the bathroom should always be a place you want to be.

Making Your Bathroom Your Favorite Room

It doesn't matter how big your bathroom is or how many people you share it with; any bathroom can become a self-care palace as long as you set it up the right way. Follow these steps and you'll never want to leave.

Keep It Minimal

No matter how the rest of your house looks, a bathroom should always be simple. Too much stuff makes any room feel smaller and bathrooms are usually the smallest room in the house anyway. Keep colors simple (like white or a light neutral) and don't overdecorate it. Lighter colors will make it feel brighter and more open.

Optimize Storage

Whether you have a lot of products around or a few, keep them organized and out of the way. Use a shower caddy or shelving unit in the shower to keep products off the floor or the sides of the tub. Switch out a standalone mirror for a medicine cabinet to keep products accessible and out of sight. Consider open shelves for additional storage, which are easy to clean and don't block airflow.

Think about Lighting

Just like you don't want to depend on overhead lighting in other parts of your house, the same goes for your bathroom. Consider getting a lighted mirror if you're worried that the light above is making you look bad in the mirror. If you have space, install sconces or alternate lighting sources so you have options. And a dimmer is your best friend, particularly if you've made baths part of your self-care routine and don't always want glaring light when you're relaxing.

Keep Supplies Handy

As you're organizing the shelves in your bathroom, keep the products you use most often accessible. This goes for your self-care supplies too. If you're taking lots of baths, for instance, keep your oils, salts, and other supplies in the bathroom in a specific place. The last thing you want to do when you're getting ready to relax is run around all the other rooms in your house.

Green It Up

Many varieties of plants, particularly those that come from tropical climates, thrive in bathrooms because of the high humidity. Keep a potted plant on a shelf or windowsill to help liven up the space and increase the quality of the air.

No Tub, No Problem

If you have a stall shower with no bathtub, you can still make your bathroom into a self-care enclave. Look for a shower stool, which you can sit on while the water is running and still get aromatherapy and relaxation benefits like you would from a bath.

Game Changers

Sometimes you can only do so much to improve the actual space of your bathroom. In those cases, upgrading some products and making minor tweaks can still give you the same effect.

Better Towels

Like sheets, upgrading your towels is a small change with a big payoff. Look for plush, soft towels in solid colors in matching sets. Bigger is usually better, but a beach towel is not the same as a bathroom towel.

Fancy Soap

Assuming you have hand soap in your bathroom (if you don't, go get some right now), getting a fancy version is a relatively small upgrade that will make you feel incredible. Instead of one with a clinical, soapy fragrance, a hand soap that has natural ingredients and essential oils will make your hands smell great, and the scent will linger in the air once you're done washing.

Diffuse, Don't Cover

Don't forget that bathrooms serve a function beyond self-care. Instead of keeping a can of air freshener on the back of the toilet, or worse, like a matchbook, get an essential oil diffuser that will consistently fill the air with a good scent. It will make less-than-pleasant smells dissipate faster and keep everything feeling clean.

Shower Curtain

In many bathrooms, the shower curtain is the unavoidable focal point. Choose a shower curtain that complements the colors of the walls (always go for lighter colors) and that you can change out or wash easily. Cloth curtains are an inexpensive way to make your bathroom look much nicer, and you can change out clear liners whenever they get dirty (which they do).

A Bathtub Caddy

If taking baths is part of your self-care practice, you're probably going to have supplies. A bathtub caddy can help keep everything in one place, like the salts or oils you put in the water, the soap you use to clean off, and even your book if you need something to do while you're soaking. Keeping everything in a caddy also means you don't need to get out of the water in the middle of your relaxation time.

Bluetooth Speaker

Whether you're soaking in a bath or just rushing through your morning shower, having a speaker in the bathroom can turn the experience from boring to actually fun. Look for a waterproof Bluetooth speaker so you don't run the risk of getting water near an electrical cord, and use it to listen to whatever you want while you're self-caring.

TREAT YOUR PRODUCTS LIKE PRODUCE

One of the easiest ways to keep a bathroom clutter-free is to regularly get rid of products that you've finished or aren't using anymore. It should go without saying that you should recycle empty bottles of shampoo, body wash, and other grooming supplies as soon as they're finished, but how often do almost-empty bottles stick around your shower? If you try something and don't like it, chuck the bottle into the recycling bin right away (but rinse it out first to make sure it's actually recycled). You might not realize that most grooming products have expiration dates too. They typically last for about a year or two, but if you have a bottle of body wash sticking around that you haven't touched in a while, you're probably not going to use it even if it hasn't expired yet. Don't keep things around for rainy days: The less you use it, the less likely you are to ever touch it again.

HOUSEPLANTS MAKE EVERYTHING BETTER

For a refresher on why interacting with nature can be considered self-care, turn back to the section on forest bathing. It all sounds great, right? But the reality is that the average person spends 93 percent of their time indoors, and finding time to go for a 2-hour forest bath, much less finding an accessible forest, is not always feasible. Most people simply don't have the time.

You might be one of those people and that's okay. You can still get some of the same benefits as a forest bath from the comfort of your home. It's because those same phytoncides that decrease your blood pressure, relieve stress, and boost your immune system are produced by every plant, not just the ones outside.

The obvious solution here is getting a houseplant. Bringing a bit of nature into your house is easy and can instantly brighten a space, not to mention relax you and make you healthier. Studies have shown that interacting with and caring for houseplants has a similar relaxation and de-stressing quality as spending time with them in nature. They work to purify the air inside, and they may even boost cognitive function. Energetically, having other living things in your home increases positive energy and helps calm frantic energy that you bring home with you.

The problem is caring for them. Like all living things, plants need basics to thrive, and you won't always know exactly what's going on, but with practice and patience, anyone can help them thrive.

The Best Plants for Black Thumbs

You don't have to be a master gardener to keep plants around. Certain plants, like the following, are decidedly hard to kill, which is why they pair perfectly with black thumbs.

Succulents
You've probably noticed these plants because they are everywhere these days: in flower shops, coffee spots, and your cool friend's house. That's because they look beautiful but don't require much care. Most of them come from hot, dry climates where water is scarce, so they store water inside and don't need to be doted on. They thrive in bright, warm light.

Snake Plants
These plants are also called "mother-in-law's tongue" because they're long and spiky like swords. They thrive in bright light but are also cool with low light, which makes them exceptional houseplants if you don't get much natural light. They love being watered but are fine if you forget. They grow tall, so you may need to repot them if they grow too much.

Pothos
These dramatic climbing plants are made to be hung in a window or left to grow over the side of a bookshelf. They root easily and grow fast in all different kinds of light, but do need water on a consistent basis. The leaves grow large and speckled, but if you notice brown leaves it's an indication it's thirsty.

Spider Plant

Spider plants are known for their long, spindly leaves that grow over the side of pots. They are all about drama and easily grow with little water and light. As they mature, they sometimes form offshoots that can be cut and repotted. A spider plant could last years and with proper care will multiply into a colony.

Cacti

Like succulents, cacti are desert plants so are perfect if you aren't great at remembering to water. They need very little except for bright sunlight, so put them in a window or on a balcony where they can grow tall. They're truly the plant dummy's dream because they seem to do best when you don't do anything at all.

Bamboo

You've probably seen bamboo in offices and malls; that's because these hearty plants do well in even the worst conditions. Bamboo grows in both bright and low light, doesn't need a lot of water, and the air quality doesn't matter. It's a great plant to keep on your desk at work or in a dimly lit bedroom.

Aloe

Aloe plants are succulents, so they don't need much water but do prefer bright light. Keep a potted aloe on the windowsill of your kitchen or somewhere close by. The sap inside the leaves is a powerful burn healer and skin moisturizer so comes in handy any time you might burn yourself taking something out of the oven.

How to Keep a Plant Alive

Caring for plants isn't as hard as it seems. They just need the same things you do and a little patience.

Water

Like all living things, plants need water in order to survive, even hearty plants like succulents and cacti. Water your plants regularly (once a week is a good place to start) and soak the soil in each pot thoroughly in a circular motion. If water starts running out the bottom of the pot, stop. A good rule is if the plant's leaves turn yellow, it's overwatered, and if they turn brown, it needs more.

Light

Plants depend on light for photosynthesis, the process in which they turn chlorophyll to food. This means that even if a plant does well in "low light," it still needs some in order to live. Low light does not mean complete darkness. Most plants will come with an instruction card when you buy them that tells you what kind of light they need. Direct light means they do well in a window, indirect light means they do well on a bookshelf or table, and low light means they're good for a darker room that still has a window.

Air

Just like humans, plants need to breathe. Airflow is important when it comes to plants since putting them in a closed-off space with little air circulation won't help them grow. Keep your room well ventilated with open windows or fans, or, better yet, keep them outside on a porch or balcony.

Temperature

Like with airflow, many plants are sensitive to temperature. Pay particular attention to vents and heaters, which may not always be on but could be detrimental to plants when they are. For instance, a plant might thrive sitting on a radiator during the summer, but once it kicks on when it gets cold, it could scorch and kill the plant.

Pot

The size of the pot is important for any houseplant. If it's too big, the plant has to work harder to leech nutrients from the soil; if it's too small, the plant has nowhere to grow. When you buy a plant, ask someone at the store what the best pot size is for that particular plant. Always make sure the pot has a drainage hole in the bottom so extra water doesn't soak and kill the roots (get a saucer to avoid mess).

Soil

When you're choosing soil for houseplants, always look for soil specific to potted plants. It will have dense nutrients specifically formulated for contained environments like pots. Don't try to save money by digging up soil from the park down the street. Bagged soil is usually sterilized against pests and germs that could not only kill your plants but infest your house.

IS THERE SUCH A THING AS TOO MANY PLANTS?

Having one plant in your home can make a huge difference, but is it possible to go overboard? Yes and no. Studies have shown that plants thrive in a plant-rich environment. They regulate the humidity in the air, and having other plants around can help them each thrive even more. They have also been shown to create a kind of mini-ecosystem when grouped together. However, too much clutter can make plants hard to care for. Pests have an easier time jumping from plant to plant, and dusty leaves can mean plants have a harder time getting the sunlight they need.

CANDLES: WHY YOU SHOULD LIGHT UP

It's a common self-care trope: A lady luxuriating in a bubble bath, glass of wine in hand, soft music playing, surrounded by the flickering light of candles. It's such a common idea that it's next to impossible to think of a relaxing bath without this picture coming to mind. And when you see it in movies or on TV, it's almost always a woman. This cliché has done more than almost anything else to create the idea that candles are feminine. They're not. Candles are totally rad and if you really think about it, pretty damn masculine. Honestly, what could be more dude-friendly than setting something on fire?

You'll be hard-pressed to find something that instantly changes the vibe of a room or environment like a candle. The fire itself has a soothing effect, the flickering light signals relaxation, and specific scents have actual effects on your brain. It's not just all in your head either. Scented candles have real, measurable effects on your body, and that's why they're a useful and common aromatherapy tool.

How Does Aromatherapy Work?

Aromatherapy is built upon the idea that specific scents create reactions in your brain. It's been scientifically proven that the olfactory receptors in your nose have direct links to your brain. By using brain mapping, scientists have found that specific scents cause certain parts of your brain to react. Lavender, for instance, has an actual effect on your brain's theta waves, which are responsible for relaxation and sleepiness. Other scents, when inhaled, have different effects like energizing, focus, or de-stressing. Science has also proven that scent is closely tied to memory, which is why certain scents sometimes take you back to previous moments in your life that you might have forgotten.

But Why Candles?

Simple. The combination of heat and the essential oils in the candle's wax diffuse the scents into the air quickly and effectively. It's called the candle's "hot throw," which is how quickly a space becomes infused with scent. High-quality candles have a high hot throw, which means that they don't even have to stay lit for very long for the smell to circulate.

Learning to use certain scents to manipulate your brain takes some trial and error, but is easy. The first step is to find a scent you like. You don't need to know what its aromatherapeutic properties are, just that you like the way it smells. Light it when you're alone and see how you respond. Do you feel chilled out? Do you feel more focused? Understanding how the smell makes you feel will help you decide how to use it. Sometimes candles will even have moods or places on the label to guide you (like "relax" or "fireplace"). Most importantly, don't overthink it. Choose a candle you like enough to use often.

There is literally no bad time to use a candle. Light one while you're meditating or about to go to sleep (but blow it out before you go to bed). Light a candle before you have a visitor over or after you've smudged your house. Light one in your kitchen after you do the dishes to signal that your kitchen is clean. And yes, you can even light one in your bathroom while you're taking a bath. You don't have to have a special occasion to light a candle—and they should be used often—but it does help to always have one burning when you have company if for no other reason than to just make your house smell better.

Best Candle Scents for Men

Choosing the right candle for you is a personal experience, but if you're new to scents, look for some of these to get started.

Sandalwood
This natural wood has a smoky and subtle sweetness, like a bonfire in the middle of the desert.

Pine
It's like having a Christmas tree in your house all year round and makes your house a thousand times cozier in an instant.

Patchouli
This herbal scent is earthy and musky and in its pure form can be overwhelming to some people. It's usually mixed with other botanical and woody scents.

Palo Santo
Just like when it's used for smudging, the scent of palo santo is smoky and purifying, but also lends an air of mystery.

Neroli
A citrus scent, it's a bit subtler than orange or lemon but still energizing. It adds a freshness to the air that makes you think of summer.

Vetiver
This herb smells sharp and green like the first day of spring. Mixed with other herbal plant scents, it creates a crispness that smells fresh and clean without being astringent.

Leather
Unlike woods and musks, leather scents aren't earthy, but they're still warm and cozy. They're ideal for cold winter months and are usually mixed with other cozy notes.

Candle Safety for the Pyrophobic

If lighting a candle in your house freaks you out, there are a few simple steps to burning one safely.

Keep the Wick Trimmed
Making sure the wick isn't too long will keep the flame low and smoke to a minimum. Trim the wick down with a trimmer or pair of scissors after every use.

Keep It in the Open
Never burn a candle near possibly flammable things like papers, books, plants, or clothes. Keep it on an open table or counter.

Never Leave It Unattended
Most candles come in containers, but they can still fall over or spill out. Never leave the room with a candle still burning or burn it in a place you can't see easily.

Always Stay Awake
If you light a candle to help you relax or fall asleep, don't leave it burning through the night. Let the scent do its job to relax you but blow it out before you go to bed.

Use a Snuffer

Blowing out candles is quick, but if you're concerned about melted wax flying everywhere, use a candlesnuffer. It helps extinguish candles without mess.

SET THE MOOD WITH SCENT

Candles aren't just for making your place smell good or covering up bad odors. The power of aromatherapy lies in its ability to change your emotions or mood. If you're trying to create a certain vibe, like if you have a date coming over or your in-laws are visiting, you can use candles to actually change how they (and you) perceive the space. These are just some examples:

- **Calm and relaxed:** Use candles with ingredients like lavender and eucalyptus to create a calm, spa-like atmosphere.
- **Clean and bright:** Burning a candle with citrus notes like lemon, bergamot, or neroli signals to your nose that the place is fresh and clean.
- **Cozy and welcoming:** Wintery notes like cinnamon, wood, and leather give a cozy depth to the air and make it feel warm and inviting (like you have a fireplace, even if you don't).
- **Casual and breezy:** Herbal notes like vetiver, rosemary, basil, and other green plants can make even a windowless space feel open and breezy and can even make a room feel more open and spacious.
- **Sexy and mysterious:** Use a candle with exotic notes like frankincense, sandalwood, and palo santo to create a smoky, sensual vibe to signal you're ready to get down to business.

HOW TO CREATE A SCENT STORY

Men wear cologne for a lot of reasons: to make themselves feel sexier, give themselves some extra swagger, attract other people, or cover up something that doesn't smell so great. Most men treat cologne as the final step in their grooming routine, like a cherry on top of a sundae. A spritz of cologne here and there has a remarkable ability to completely transform your mood and cover up a variety of evils.

The thing is, most guys' experience with fragrance ends there. They don't think about all the other ways fragrance affects their lives and, in particular, their homes. You might not think how your home smells matters, but it does. You've definitely been to someone's house before where you've walked in and immediately thought that something didn't quite smell right. Walking into a funky-smelling space is a hard feeling to shake, even if eventually you get used to it. Now think about a time you've walked into someone's home and it smelled amazing. There's a feeling associated with that too, and it's definitely not bad. Wouldn't you rather be the person whose house smells good?

There has been a lot of discussion in this book about the benefits of aromatherapy, and it's all true. You can use smell to change your mood and activate certain parts of your brain. The problem is that when your home smells bad, it's a bit like living in the monkey cage. Eventually you get used to the smell and it doesn't affect you anymore. At least you think it doesn't. If it's been established that certain smells can alter your mood, can you imagine being in a place where the bad smells are consistently bringing you down? If your home has a funk, it could be. You might not even notice it till you make a few changes.

On top of all that, good smells welcome visitors and invite positivity. They also have the power to cover up a lot of things. If you frantically clean your place before someone comes over, shoving dirty clothes in the hamper and loading the dishwasher with dishes, lingering smells can betray you. If your home smells great, guests are much less likely to notice when things are dirty. That should be reason enough.

What to Use

There is an entire toolbox of options to create a well-scented and happy-feeling home. What you choose comes down to preference.

Candles

Scented candles are the valedictorian of the home scent world, but they aren't the end-all-be-all. Turn back to the previous section for a refresher on why they're good and how to use them.

Incense

People discount incense because of its associations with college town head shops and stuffy church services, but you shouldn't! Nothing fills a space with fragrance quicker or better than a quick hit of incense. Not only is it a great conversation starter but it also instantly makes your place seem mysterious and interesting.

Diffusers

Fans of diffusers say they are better and safer than candles, but they're not for everyone. Some diffusers use natural reeds stuck in essential oils to draw the fragrance into the air. Others use small flames to heat liquid or can even be plugged into a wall outlet.

They're usually subtler, and instead of scenting the air quickly like a candle, they offer a constant background smell like white noise.

Room Sprays

Think of a room spray like cologne for your house: You spray it into the air and the scent lingers. But don't think you can use cologne to the same effect. Wearable fragrance, like cologne, is formulated to sit on your skin and react to its warmth. Room sprays, however, have lighter molecules that stay suspended in air longer and don't need heat to stay fragrant.

Linen Sprays

You might know linen spray by another name: Febreze. But unlike the famous odor killer, a high-end linen spray won't leave your couch or sheets smelling like new-car smell. Using a linen spray with essential oils can give you additional aromatherapy benefits too. Spray a lavender spray on your sheets and pillows for better sleep, for instance, or eucalyptus spray on the place your dog always sleeps on your couch to neutralize the odor.

Drawer Sachets

Keeping a scented sachet in your dresser drawers and closet can not only keep your clothes smelling fresh, but can ward off pests like moths too. Closed spaces trap odor and moisture, which is why your sweaters sometimes have a musty smell when you get them out of storage in the fall. Scenting your drawers keeps that under control.

How to Create a Signature Scent

Just like choosing a cologne, deciding on how your house should smell takes some thought. You want people to remember it once they leave—in a good way.

Think about the Mood You Want to Set

The same principles of aromatherapy go into scenting your home as other areas of self-care. If you want to create a relaxing, calm atmosphere for instance, use notes like lavender to increase chill vibes. Citrus scents are energizing and usually make things smell clean, where scents like wood and smoke create a cozy, warm ambience.

Mix Different Products

When conceptualizing your scent story, don't feel like you have to stick to just one thing. Mix products like candles and incense to create layers of discovery. Place different tools in different rooms to keep people guessing. And remember, stronger isn't always better.

Get Inspired by Nature

Most men don't gravitate toward sweet or food-inspired scents in the first place, but when in doubt look to nature. Fragrances that come from trees, plants, and other natural substances generally smell better in larger areas like homes. Think about how great your house smells when you have a Christmas tree up; a pine-scented candle can give you the same effect without your needing to clean up the needles afterward.

Better Yet, Use Living Things

Supplement your natural-scented candles and diffusers with the real thing for extra power. Bring in fresh flowers or fragrant plants to make the good smells more layered and more realistic than you could ever get with a candle alone. Think of them as complementing the scent, not competing with it, and choose plants that are similar to the notes found in the candle or diffuser you're using.

Pick a Through Line

When you start delving into the world of home scents, it's easy to go overboard. Instead of throwing everything at the wall and seeing what sticks (or, in this case, smells good), pick a theme and build up on it. Choose multiple products that all have the same note. For instance, if you like wood scents, pick a few different candles that all have sandalwood in them, and place them in different rooms of the house. It will keep the scent layers from fighting each other.

Keep It Clean

You're doing all this work to make your house smell great, so you don't want other things competing with it, do you? Household scents can overpower even the strongest candle without you knowing it. Always empty the trash, clear the sink of dirty dishes, and stow away dirty laundry if you want your good smells to take center stage.

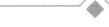

DON'T STICK TO JUST ONE

Scent pros do something you probably don't: They use different scents in different rooms of their houses. It's easier than you might think. First, find a few different scents that work well together and then place them strategically throughout the house like this:

- **Foyer or front door:** Have a candle or diffuser that smells inviting, like something with vanilla or spices to draw people into your home.
- **Kitchen:** Go for freshness like citrus or green herbals to signal that your place is clean.

- **Living room:** Light up a candle with cozy notes like pine or sandalwood to recall a crackling fire and invite people to relax.
- **Bathroom:** Keep a diffuser tucked away with a scent of eucalyptus or sage to make the space feel open and chill.
- **Bedroom:** If you're expecting a little hanky-panky, choose a sexy scent like frankincense, and if you just want to chill out and sleep, opt for something with lavender.

INDEX

Index

ABOUT THE AUTHOR

Garrett Munce is a writer and editor specializing in men's grooming, beauty, style, and wellness. He is the grooming editor for *Esquire* and *Men's Health*, and was previously grooming director and senior fashion editor at *GQ*. With over a decade in editorial experience, he has also contributed to *Town & Country*, *W*, *Teen Vogue*, *New York* magazine, *Refinery29*, *Gear Patrol*, and more. He also serves as editor-at-large for the men's beauty site *Very Good Light*. He lives in Brooklyn with his husband, their naughty pug, and more skincare products than he knows what to do with.